36 A DAY!

...36+ children a day diagnosed with cancer

Judy A. Dees

First published by Amazon Create Space July 2016

ISBN: 13:978-1533098535

Library of Congress Control Number

Printed in the United States of America

1. Children's health 2. Cancer 3. Chemical illness 4. Dangers of fragrances

TABLE OF CONTENTS

DEDICATION

First, as always, to the One who knew me before I was born and chose my creation; the One who never left me in the worst times of my life; the One who gave me hope when I had no hope; the One who was my spiritual husband and best friend the many years I was alone; the One who is the Maker of Heaven and Earth; the One who walked with me through the valley of the shadow of death and saved my life; and the One who pulled me out of the mire and saved my soul—the one true Lord God Almighty.

Second, to all children and teens in the world. I cannot physically see you, but spiritually I can. My heart is ever for you. I believe in each one of you. Father God saw fit for you to be born, so He has a plan for you—a plan to give you hope and a future, NOT plans to harm you. So if you are in harm's way, KNOW this is not of God and not His plan for you.

This book is about the harm chemicals will inflict upon you. I pray your caregivers have and use this book. I pray they pass it on to you to use with your future family.

This is an important book for you, but the most important book, forever, is God's book, the Bible. It will tell you all you need to know in this life here on earth (70-80 years) and will prepare you for Eternity (thousands of years). Your decision to accept or reject God's son Jesus is the most important decision you will EVER make.

Go forth, Sons and Daughters of mankind. Make choices in your breathing, eating, and drinking—and in your soul—that will bring you health and life.

Third, I wish to dedicate this book to ones whose lives have been taken by cancer. In my circle were my grandmother Mary Bruce, my mother Hazel Anderson, my brother Woodrow Anderson Jr., my niece Tess Anderson, my friend Dianne McMichael, and numerous other relatives and friends.

INTRODUCTION

36 a day!

36 children a day!

36 children a day diagnosed with cancer!

Since national TV announced this statistic in late 2010, I have not rested. In that same year, St. Jude Children's Research Hospital in Memphis, Tennessee, cited (in a letter to contributors) treatment of 5,700 children with cancer. Thousands more would develop cancer that year. My heart ached for them. Imagine how these children and parents hurt! It is past time to come to the aid of our children. What else must they endure? Our most precious gifts from God and our nation's most valuable assets—children—are neglected, abused, discarded, abducted, and now given to all kinds of illnesses, which should be unnatural for childhood.

Several years ago, I accompanied my daughter and grandson to Arkansas Children's Hospital. As we sat in the asthma clinic waiting room, I looked around. Here was my young grandson with his inhaler. Across the room sat a child who wore a protective mask. Two or three babies with breathing problems cried loud and long. Other children coughed continuously. I had been ill for years with respiratory problems, so I knew how they felt. My heart felt it could burst! Tears flooded my eyes. My mission in life became clear: continue to help children. No longer a classroom teacher (because of this illness), I would always be a teacher.

I began to share and teach what I had learned. Everyone who crossed my path heard about the harmful chemicals in our food, drink, and air. Almost every day for years now, I've shared my own story of illness and road to recovery. Since this TV announcement about childhood cancer and recent statistics about large asthma/allergy increases, a broader goal emerged for me: reach every possible parent and child caregiver with this message.

Information in *36 A DAY!* is not all inclusive. It is simply a basic guide to improve your child's (and family's) health. It could possibly prevent your child being 1 of the 36+ a day diagnosed with cancer or other diseases caused by toxic food, drink, and air consumption.

My desire is to help others (especially children) avoid going through what I went through—or worse. I am an ordinary person who became very ill for many years. Until age 45, I had been strong and fairly healthy, although I had some allergies. I was sick two to four times a year. Later, my state of being was that of being sick most of the time. It took over 15 years from the time I lost my health to the time I regained much of it. There are many treatments available for illness; my contention is that WE SHOULD AIM FOR PREVENTION of illness.

After discovering the causes of my own chronic illness (chemicals), I began to make changes in lifestyle. With continual improvement, today I am NOT a person who has bad allergies or asthma. I seldom get sick and am NOT confined to my home as was the case for about eight years.

2

Still learning and changing! In the years of research which aided my recovery, I noticed that many of the same chemicals (especially fragrances) that caused me problems contained carcinogens and caused respiratory and central nervous system issues. The proverbial "light bulb" flashed! Like 2 + 2 + 2 = 6, SO carcinogen + carcinogen+ carcinogen = cancer! ALL THE HARMFUL CHEMICALS WE BREATHE, EAT, and DRINK MUST BE STRONG CONTRIBUTORS TO THE CANCER, ALLERGY, ASTHMA, and OTHER ILLNESSES THAT ARE ON THE RISE! In this book, I want to share with you, parents and caregivers of children, what I've learned (years of research) and experienced. I have lived the horror of chemically induced illness—and, praise God, survived.

*See "MY STORY" at the end of PART I.

Dr. Max Gerson was a top authority in the study of natural treatment of cancer. He reported that in the 1940's, 1 in 16 people had cancer. In 2006, it was 1 in 3, nearing 1 in 2.[i]

Many of you have lost beloved family or friends to the dread disease cancer. Perhaps you have experienced that pain of loss. If not, to some degree, you might have felt other families' fears or shared their pain. Most victims were probably adults. But how many have experienced the great loss of a child to cancer?

Can you imagine what these children must suffer, even if they survive? The fear. The pain. Children should be enjoying childhood with few cares, instead of having the weight of cancer on their shoulders. A head full of hair should shine bright and healthy — not be dry, brittle, or even bald from chemotherapy. (A friend who works at a hospital told me if any chemo is spilled, they have to shut down the area to clean, and if any gets on their skin, it burns badly. Imagine what it does to the insides of a person.) Their skin should be soft and smooth rather than leathery, calloused, and blistered (that hurts with touch) from radiation. Being sick and nauseous should be caused by a virus or from eating too much birthday cake — not from cancer treatments. Unless sick children know of Heaven, where is hope?

A visitor to my (former) store (Mr. B's Ice Cream & Deli in Branson, MO) told about her 44-year-old son who died from lung cancer. He was not a smoker. She was convinced that the fast foods he ate and the pollution in the air killed him. I've known many adults who died of cancer; several smoked or worked in chemical environments. (I knew well two people who had Parkinson's disease which is also connected to chemicals, especially pesticides. One used a fly pesticide spray at her front door entrance for about ten years; the other was an art teach of many years.)

Every child has the right to breathe clean air — not polluted, toxic air. Food choices may be made, but air quality may not. If one person in a room uses a fragranced product, everyone in that room has to breathe the chemicals in the fragrance for it contains VOC's (volatile organic compounds) which are very difficult to contain or restrict. If one mist spray is emitted by a fragrance deodorizer, everyone in the room breathes it. The same is true of one puff of cigarette smoke. What are YOU making those around you breathe? It is an uninformed person who pollutes the air of others because they think it smells or tastes good or masks their lack of personal hygiene.

A loving parent, grandparent, or teacher/caregiver will pursue what is best for the children in his or her life. Children depend on these important people to protect and nourish them. A hard question: Are you nourishing OR harming the children in your life?

QUICK START FOR HEALTHIER LIVING
SHORT LIST/SUMMARY

1. Get rid of chemically fragranced products, especially plug-in deodorizers. If you must have fragrances, use real essential oils (found mainly in health food stores). Use lemons, limes, oranges, cinnamon, or vanilla. Use fragrance-free (FF) products.

2. Avoid breathing fragrances, smoke, exhaust, and other toxic chemicals and their fumes. Dishwashing soaps can be very toxic. The fragranced ones expel the harmful chemicals throughout your home. They even stick to the dishes on which you place your family's food so are being eaten as well.

3. Consider what you eat and drink. Make healthier choices. Avoid a lifestyle of fast and processed foods or snack foods. Eat more fresh vegetables, fruits, and whole grains. Organic is best. Drink mainly purified or healthier water; avoid (or limit greatly) sweet, chemical drinks, especially the diet drinks.

4. Use natural products for your cleaning and deodorizing needs: vinegar, baking soda, essential oils, lemons, limes, oranges, cinnamon, or vanilla. Dr. Bronner's Sal Suds at health food stores is one of my favorites.

5. Check your detergents and soaps. Since the skin is the body's largest organ, detergents and soaps are very important. All Free is the #1 recommended by dermatologists, pediatricians, and allergists; however, other fragrance-free detergents are available and

better than the strongly scented ones. Use no fabric softener, or put vinegar or baking soda in the final rinse cycle. Some FF or unscented soaps are available, especially at health food stores. Watch unscented products! They may contain a fragrance. *Unscented* means no fragrance was added; some ingredients may be scented, however.

6. Do not be overwhelmed! Read the next pages and see simple solutions. You can make a BIG difference in the health of your family. The way to eat an elephant is one bite at a time; begin with one thing at a time.

PART I: 36 A DAY!

Where are your children the majority of each day? School? Daycare? Home? Most are at school 8-10 hours a day. Most are at home 14-16 hours a day. Does it make sense for these two places to be as environmentally safe as possible for them? If you worked to get home and school as fragrance / chemical free as possible, your children's health and lives would benefit greatly. Benefits are from the inside out. Chemical free is the ideal environment for children. Then when they have to be in other toxic environments, their bodies will not be as ravaged. They will be strong enough to fight pollutants to which they are exposed.

Where does a family begin? FIRST, clean up your home. SECOND, ask schools to do the same. Work with other parents, relatives, and churches. Some will want nothing to do with any change or clean up; merely continue your pursuit of a healthier environment for YOUR children. In many years of sharing this information or my story, I've noticed that some listen and some don't. However, facts and a personal testimony speak the truth about harmful chemicals.

Let's get busy! Two basic steps assure your success: (1) Identify problem areas. (2) Remove them and replace with healthier choices.

STEP 1: IDENTIFY PROBLEM AREAS.

Identify the foods and drinks you consume that contain chemicals, additives, and preservatives. Very important: READ THE LABELS!! Identify the fragranced, chemical products your family uses. Smell the products. If your olfactory senses are not impaired from continual exposure to fragrances, "sniff-out" culprits. If they are damaged, check the label to see if the product contains fragrance. Guess what? The shocking truth is that the contents of the fragrance itself are not labeled. Trade Secret, the perfume industry calls it. If they labeled their products, no one would buy them because of the toxic contents.[ii] Later in this book (PART II: FYI), I will list some of the contents, and you will see the reasons they are not identified. I do know that most fragrances contain harmful — even toxic — chemicals. Who would buy these fragranced products if the contents were revealed?

STEP 2: REMOVE THEM!

Get rid of harmful products and replace with healthier ones! Call or write companies whose products you like and use. Ask that they quit using harmful chemicals and quit adding cheap, toxic fragrances and additives to these items. Demand that they label and reveal any potentially harmful chemicals. Stop buying their unsafe products, and see if THAT gets their attention.   Better yet, find healthy alternatives. (See PART II: FYI)

Most foods have labels; therefore, choices are made to eat or not eat them. So let's focus first on air that is breathed. Fragrances and chemicals offer no choice as their VOC (volatile organic compound) composition makes them hard to confine; they permeate their surroundings. Their ingredients are often not labeled. In all cases, identify products to which your child is most exposed.

AIR CHILDREN BREATHE —
FRAGRANCED PRODUCTS

I targeted fragrances first because most people do not realize that chemical FRAGRANCES ARE TOXIC.[iii] Not only are they toxic (U.S. Postal Service labels them hazardous.), but also they do not dissipate rapidly. By nature, fragrances adhere to skin, hair, and other surfaces; they are not easily removed because of petroleum and pesticide contents. FRAGRANCES ARE PERHAPS THE MOST WIDESPREAD AND DECEPTIVE CHEMICALS IN USE. Their VOC composition causes them to permeate the environment. Every nearby lung, sinus, and skin surface inhales or absorbs the toxins.[iv]

PERSONAL CARE PRODUCTS

Perfumes and Colognes

Obviously, these are fragrances. (See PART II: FYI   for a partial list of ingredients found in fragrances; see reasons for its environmental name Sweet Poison.) The Fragrance Industry lists 2,993 materials used in fragrance compounds in 2011.[v] I could not pronounce over half the ingredients, and only a few would I put on my body or want to breathe.

If anyone in your household wears this Sweet Poison— even if you love the smell—all in the household are affected just by breathing it. Allergies and sinuses can be irritated; asthma may be triggered or developed. Undesirable behavior and emotions may surface. Depression and headaches often increase. Cancer or other illnesses are seeded. Chemical fragrances could be a close third in pollution to exhaust fumes and cigarette smoke![vi]

Alternatives: essential oils. Mix essential oils with water as a spray, or mix with coconut oil or jojoba oil as a cream.

Shampoos, Hair Conditioners, Hair Gels & Sprays

A young lady who worked at my store had hair that looked and felt like straw. Her hair products were very strong. She started using an organic FF (fragrance-free) shampoo. After a few weeks, she ran in one day. "Judy, my hair has quit falling out! And look how shiny and soft it is!" Most hair products contain fragrances, as well as other harmful chemicals. This residue is absorbed by or adheres to the hair shaft and follicles. It is stored dangerously close to the brain.[vii] READ THE LABELS. Note fragrances (parfums), anything with *propyl,* and chemicals you cannot pronounce or with which you are not familiar. They are harmful.

Alternatives: Health food stores have healthier gels and hairsprays. They have shampoos/conditioners that contain essential oils or that are fragrance free. (See PART II: FYI for homemade soda wash/vinegar rinse.)

Body Soaps & Lotions

Anything rubbed onto the skin goes into the bloodstream, thus into the body (similar to nicotine and birth control patches). Keep in mind that all these products, if fragrant, emit harmful toxins into the air.

Alternatives: I try to put nothing on my skin that I cannot eat: Coconut, olive, or almond oils are my favorites and great as lotions. Dr. Bronner, Kiss My Face, Zum, and others natural brands have great soaps. Look for soaps and lotions with less harsh ingredients — and fragrance free or made with essential oils. Target stocks Method Go Naked soaps. Their scented soaps (and other Method products), however, contain the chemical fragrances.

Make-Up & Cosmetics

Most facial cosmetics are composed of products a person would never consider using. [viii] Yet, here they are, soaking into women's faces! Women (and some men) breathe the strong fragrances all day long then complain of headaches, depression, or fatigue. Some women say they don't wear fragrance because it bothers them, yet they are wearing make-up that smells strongly of fragrance. !!!??? As children snuggle close to Mom or Dad, they get it all over themselves; if they kiss Mom, they are, in essence, "eating" it, too! The phthalates in cosmetics are being studied because some researchers think they are a big cause of sterility or problems in male children.[ix] Europe, unlike America, strongly regulates the ingredients in personal care products.

Alternatives: Bare Minerals, Mineral Fusion, and other brands at health food stores seem to be the best offered. How about no base on the face? Accent the eyes. I've used no base for over 15 years. My face is in much better condition, and I can smile without cracking my face.

Sunscreen

Sunscreen, too, contains harmful chemicals and fragrances — and it's most difficult to remove. The smell lingers through many baths and much laundering. Children at daycare have to endure this toxin in exchange for 15 minutes of outside play. Have parents and teachers forgotten children's great need for sunlight?

Alternatives: Check environmental groups like EWG (Environmental Working Group) for a list of safer sunscreens. (Since they came out with it a few years ago, the list has grown tremendously!) Or, why not let the children absorb some good Vitamin D from the sun? Schedule recess early in the day. Wear T shirts when swimming. Put hats or safer sunscreen on the head.

HOUSEHOLD AND CLEANING PRODUCTS

Laundry Detergents & Fabric Softeners

These are major! Like your body soaps, they cover your body; their fragrant, chemical residue is in the fiber of the clothes you wear. Not only are you breathing all day (clothing) and night (bedding, pajamas) their toxic fragrances, but also they are soaking into your skin and going through the bloodstream to all parts of the body. [x] Research your brand! Don't buy the cheapest brand available unless it is the best. The extensive Canadian study (PART II: FYI) found that the two most toxic detergents are very popular brands, BOTH made by the same company. Think about fabric softeners. If fabric softener alters the fiber of clothing, what does it do to you? A class action lawsuit was recently filed against the fabric softener industry.[xi] Much information is available about its dangers (as well as dangers of fragrances).

Alternative: When I was sickest, All Free was the only detergent (besides organic) I could tolerate, and I still use it or Seventh Generation. I use absolutely no fabric softener but put vinegar in my final rinse or the fabric softener compartment. And no, my laundry doesn't smell like vinegar! Try baking soda/water paste or hydrogen peroxide on those tough spots and stains. They are natural so do have to soak a while. My daughters add a few essential oil drops to their All Free detergent to give a light, pleasant smell to their laundry.

Dish & Dishwasher Detergents

These contain fragrances. If it's not enough that we ingest these toxins through our lungs, sinuses, and skin, now we eat fragrances. The fragrant residue adheres to the dishes on which we eat so we eat it along with our food. How crazy is this? In addition, when dishwasher detergent is heated to steam vapor temperature, the fragrance remains for hours, and your family breathes it as they sleep.

Alternatives: Great news! Some Walmart stores and Target carry Seventh Generation (fragrance-free, free & clear, or with essential oils) dish detergent and dishwasher detergents. Encourage your local stores to stock them! Also Target carries Method Go Naked fragrance-free products. Avoid Method's fragranced products, though, as they are made with the chemical fragrances.

Deodorizers: Plug-Ins & Wall-Mounted

These products can be more harmful than ordinary fragrance because they contain extra pesticide and propellants [xii] (See PART II: FYI). I cannot over emphasize the importance of ridding your home of these toxic, Sweet Poison devices. Besides penetrating your home's breathing space, they often emit a spray that can adhere to a nearby person. This happened to me two or three times. I had to wear the odious smell and had the ensuing headache and discomfort.

Once it affected my behavior so badly that the manager of a restaurant in which we were eating had to come to my family's table. I had gone to the restroom. As I squatted, the deodorizer mounted over the toilet sprayed; of course, I could not move! I wish I had known or thought to take off my shirt and call my family. I returned to the table, we ordered, then it began— in a matter of maybe 10 minutes. To this day, I don't remember all that happened, but I do know I became very agitated and aggressive— enough that the waitress had the manager come out. This was one of the great embarrassing moments of my life— one over which I had no control, caused by a deodorizer.

I often wonder about the behavior of children whose homes are contaminated with these toxic fragrances. Deodorizers are especially harmful for children, seniors, and people with asthma, allergies, or respiratory weakness. And they contain extra carcinogens.[xiii] Yes, they often smell good— Sweet Poison!

Alternatives: Health food stores and some department stores have small and large mist diffusers for use with essential oils and water. I also get small spray bottles and fill them with water and 10-12 drops of my favorite essential oils to use as deodorizer sprays in my house. Fruit peels, along with cinnamon or vanilla, may also be used as harmless deodorizers.

Candles

Candles add a warm glow to the home, and their Sweet Poison smell wafts throughout the house. This brings comfort and pleasure to some in the household, but it brings discomfort and pain to others—and seeds future or present illness and disease. Candles play on the aesthetics more than most fragranced products, but they are just as toxic.

Alternatives: Fragrance-free candles are available. I use my essential oil mist diffuser or my spray bottle of essential oil and water mix…then a battery or fragrance-free candle for the glow.

Disinfectants & Cleaners

These are many, with as many different smells as there are varieties. Some of the most popular are fragranced with sweet perfume or pine chemicals. Many are sprays, so the VOC's penetrate more area. Again, the fragrances are toxic, and other harmful chemicals are among the ingredients. Some literally take away a person's breath! I was outside recently, and my neighbor shot out her front door. I asked her what was wrong. She told me she'd been cleaning her bathtub with Lysol and suddenly couldn't breathe. One day I was volunteering at a local charity in the cafeteria and realized I could hardly breathe. Someone had cleaned the windows in the room next to me, and although I couldn't smell it, the fumes were affecting me.

Alternative: Vinegar is an age-old, safe disinfectant. Yale-New Haven Hospital uses it as a hospital disinfectant.[xiv] I've used it for years! Dr. Bronner's Sal Suds (at health stores) is a favorite of mine—and it smells of pine (so no need for Pine Sol). Lemon and baking soda are natural cleaners, too.

AIR CHILDREN BREATHE – HARSH CHEMICALS

Cleaning Products

Bleach or other cleaning products must be used at times when a natural cleaner will not cut the grease or stain on a floor or bathtub. Just don't use them often. Avoid breathing the harmful fumes after use. (Open a window to ventilate or close a door to contain the fumes.) If the cleaner is strong enough to remove grime, it must be a strong chemical.

Alternative: Make a baking soda/water paste. Apply to grime or grease. Soak one to several hours (especially the oven). Scrub gently and rinse. Also use lemon juice or vinegar applications. Health stores have healthier cleaning products, as well.

Pesticides and Insecticides

There might be a time when these toxic chemicals have to be used, but try to avoid them. Pesticides and insecticides greatly affect the body, especially the central nervous system. These chemicals are being linked to many illnesses like Parkinson's and Alzheimer's.[xv]

Although some have become ill and a few have died from having their homes sprayed [xvi], others have their homes or businesses sprayed three to four times a year, even monthly. I used to do that—before multiple chemical sensitivities. I have not had my house sprayed in over 20 years, and my food business of nine years saw no sprays. There was no pest problem at either place. Floors were kept clean, and

Tom's glue boards were used. I occasionally used a contained chemical for ants, Terro.

Alternatives: Borax, peppermint essential oil /water spray, glue boards, cinnamon, and mop with vinegar water. Vacuum between baseboards/flooring to get insect eggs. I use lye soap, Vitamin B or garlic supplements, or oregano oil as insect repellents…not Skin So Soft.

Exhaust

Exhaust is still the major pollutant in our country, according to authorities.[xvii] Many environmentalists think fragrance runs a close second or third! [xviii] Exhaust contains particulates of carbon monoxide, nitrogen dioxide, dinitrogen oxide, sulphur dioxide, benzene, formaldehyde, polycyclic hydrocarbons, and carbon dioxide (Green Living Tips). It is a respiratory danger for anyone, especially those with asthma, allergies, skin sensitivities, and respiratory problems.

Death can be the result of a person being in an enclosed area with a running vehicle— carbon monoxide poisoning. Is it not shocking that many cities construct their hiking and biking trails along a busy highway or interstate? Lungs of the exercisers are wide open for all that exhaust pollution!

Alternative: Try to buy vehicles with inside/outside air. This helps filter some of the exhaust that comes inside your vehicle. Keep windows rolled up when traveling busy highways. Avoid walking (especially with precious babies or children) or running along busy roads.

Tobacco Smoke

This remains a top pollutant. The Surgeon General determined (a long time ago) that cigarette smoke is hazardous to one's health. Cigarette smoke may contain up to 7,000 different chemicals. Hundreds are toxic; seventy can cause cancer.[xix]A cigarette contains about 600 ingredients.[xx]

Second hand smoke is as dangerous (if not more so) to those breathing it as smoke is to a smoker. The sad concern is that children and other non-smokers have no choice about the smoke they sometimes have to breathe. Some smoker parents are considerate of other family members and go outside to smoke; others smoke inside, thus endangering all other household members.

Two situations come to mind: (1) the parent whose child has had a constant earache for weeks— and the parent continues to smoke inside the house (2) the parent whose child has had numerous sinus infections, bronchitis, or even pneumonia—and the parent still smokes inside the house.

Alternative: Quit smoking! Or at least go outside to smoke. Don't smoke in the vehicle where all have to breathe it.

Wood Smoke

If your home is heated with a wood stove or fireplace, make sure the smoke is vented out. If not, the smoke may cause respiratory infections, coughs, headaches, burning eyes, or worse. A wood furnace outside will also produce toxic smoke, so watch where the children play.

Chemical Smoke

This is often found when businesses burn their plastic or other chemical wastes rather than spending money for waste disposal pick- up. Again, it's about money and little consideration for the air others have to breathe.

Alternative: Be careful that what you burn outside is paper, wood, or biodegradable, not chemical. Do go to your city if you have a recurring "burner" nearby. What you smell might be meth!!

Construction

New construction often poses multiple health problems. Beware of strong smells and new smells. Paint, carpet, and sealers are laced with high VOC's, formaldehyde, and many other toxic chemicals.[xxi]

Alternative: Use no or low VOC paints and sealers. Check the formaldehyde level of carpets; possibly use tile or wood flooring. Air out the structure until it has finished "gassing-out."

*These next two we don't breathe, but they need to be addressed.

Immunizations

Some feel immunizations are important, even essential. Please research BEFORE you subject your children to a shot with harmful chemicals that might negatively affect them the rest of their lives. Many types of immunizations are being connected to a growing number of childhood illnesses and problems.[xxii] Immunizations ARE chemicals.

About 30 years ago, a flu shot not only gave me the flu but also kept me sick for 39 days! Do you think I ever got another flu shot? No way! Yes, I've had the flu a few times, but none made me sicker than that one flu shot.

Alternative: For several years now because I live as chemical free as possible, I seldom get the flu. When I do, I am usually sick only a few days. Getting rid of fragrances and other chemicals has freed my body and immune system to fight viruses. Try it! Maybe your child (and you) will be sick less often.

There are many natural supplements and herbs that help protect from viruses and flu. Elderberry juice, Vitamins C and D, QBC, lavender and peppermint essential oils, Thieves essential oil, oregano oil, and colloidal silver are also ones I like.

Medications
Thank God for physicians and for medicines—when they are necessary. There is a time when medication is needed. However, the problem today is that society resorts to medication at the first sign of a sniffle. Many over-the-counter meds are common household items. All of them are chemicals, some toxic chemicals.[xxiii]

Over the years, some popular meds have been recalled. Recently in the news was a common product made by a very popular company associated with babies and families. The product contained a pesticide that had been banned for years. The FDA warned them to recall; there have been many recalls and lawsuits since then.[xxiv] What was this pesticide doing in the consumable product in the first place?

Alternative: If your child's condition (cold, runny nose) isn't serious or has just begun, try this instead: (1) Eliminate all fragrances, smoke, and other chemicals from the environment. (2) Avoid sugars and other processed (junk) food. (3) Try natural supplements like Vitamin C, Vitamin D3, oregano drops, colloidal silver drops, elderberry juice, and Natural Factors lung/sinus/respiratory tablets. (4) Use homemade salt water drops in the nostrils, then blow the nose gently to remove mucous. (5) Get extra sleep and rest. (6) Drink extra amounts of pure water.

It's a good idea to have your children take good, natural multi-vitamin and mineral supplements (ones without processed sugar, high fructose corn syrup, and color additives), especially if you do not prepare nutritious meals. Even if you serve healthy foods, today's foods often do not have the minerals needed by the body because the soil has been depleted or polluted. Again, if you eliminate fragrances and other chemicals and consume foods and drinks that contain no additives, preservatives, or sugars, maybe your child won't need any medicines— chemical or natural.

FOOD CHILDREN EAT

We live in a fast-paced society. Run, run, run! Hurry, hurry, hurry! Busy, busy, busy! It is so hard, after a long day at work, to go home and cook a healthy, nutritious meal. It is much easier to get fast-food or serve a prepared meal from the grocery store. Most fast-foods and pre-packaged meals have little (or less) nutritional value and are processed foods full of preservatives, additives, or other harmful chemicals.[xxv] Thankfully, we can go to places OCCASIONALLY, when meal preparation is an impossibility. *Occasionally* is the key word here. Occasional processed chemical foods shouldn't kill a person. Some families, however, are making these foods daily menu items. Look at the lines and crowds at fast-food establishments; notice all the boxed meals in shopping carts at grocery store checkout lines.

Joyce Meyer in *New Day, New You* says, "After God created Adam and Eve, He gave them some very simple dining instructions. No, He did not tell them to freely eat fast-food, frozen pizza, or even low-fat cookies. God told Adam and Eve to eat from the garden, and we'd do well to stick to His advice. Eat the foods that come from God, in as close a state as possible to how God made them, and you can't go wrong. Only when we get corrupted by the foods made by men in laboratories and factories do we get in trouble."[xxvi]

WHERE CHILDREN EAT

Dining Out

When dining out, important considerations are menu details and the right questions. Which foods on the menu are fresh, organic, or preservative-free? Are the meats irradiated?

(1) Limit eating out. It is best to eat out no more than necessary—special occasions and vacations or when there is absolutely no time to cook or use the crock pot. It's beneficial to find a restaurant with organic or healthy, homemade foods.

(2) When you want or have to eat out, make healthier choices. Beware of fried, greasy foods; avoid processed and chemical-laden foods. Consider what your children (and you) eat. Think of the poisons or toxins swallowed. Don't deny or avoid truths about the foods you eat; merely make better choices.

(3) Choose fresh or organic salads, fruits, and vegetables rather than bagged ones that reek of preservatives. Most bagged foods have little nutritional value as they were picked some time ago, and the toxins they contain harm the body more than they benefit it. I do not eat salad at any restaurant unless I know it is free of chemicals. A few years ago, I ate salad from a "gourmet" sandwich shop. I was sick for 11 days! My colon was in excruciating pain the first three days. Why did I eat it when I could smell something on it

other than the dressing? What does it take to get a person's attention?

(4) Choose real foods over artificial foods. Try baked potatoes rather than French fries, especially the chemical, sugary fries served many places. Get real chicken pieces rather than irradiated nuggets or formations. Ask for 100% beef rather than mixtures or irradiated meats. (Some places serve burgers that are small % meat with large % fillers including ammonia.)[xxvii] Research irradiated products. I've seen exploded chickens and rotten meat, fruits, and vegetables and have no desire to be near them, let alone eat them— especially after they've been radiated to alter their state of being.

(5) Watch the breads! Find places that make (preferably) or bake their own bread. Avoid breads that become plastic-like when cold; they are full of preservatives and dough conditioners.

One customer at my store told of buying a child's burger meal. It wasn't eaten, so she decided to put it in a zip lock bag. She forgot about it then found it a few weeks later. The burger was still intact! Unbelievable! And it had a plastic-like appearance. (Could this be anything like embalming?) Another customer had just researched the bun of a fast-food establishment. According to her research, the bun had no real food in it; it was artificial and chemical products. A friend of mine bought a little packaged snack cake in October, 2009. He decided to check for himself how preserved it was. It looked the same for over three years! (More embalming?)

(6) Ask for real butter, not margarine or imitation butter spreads. Enjoy real butter; avoid overuse. Although butter contains more fat, it won't have all the chemicals of margarine. One article I read in a reputable magazine stated that margarine is one ingredient away from being plastic. I would never think of eating plastic!

(7) Make sure the meats you choose are NOT irradiated meats. Order pure cuts of meat rather than the heavily breaded, fried cuts. Healthier choices tend to be fish, chicken, and turkey; however, avoid farm-raised fish and all meats that have antibiotics and hormones added. Free range or organic (without chemicals) are the healthiest choices.

Eating at Home

Eating meals at home— if better food choices are made— will greatly improve your child's health and lessen his/her chance for cancer and other illness. The importance of READING THE LABELS cannot be overemphasized. Read labels of foods you bring into your home. Do your screening at the grocery store. Soon you'll remember which products to get and which to avoid. Make a list of foods and brand names if necessary. Know your child's weaknesses (and yours) and try to keep those foods out of the house. If food is on my shelves on in my refrigerator, I consider it "fair game."

Sugar (and high fructose corn syrup) and white flour products should be monitored or eliminated. Remember that milk and milk products can cause allergy problems for many children, joint problems for some. Sugar and flour also seem to affect allergies and behavior.[xxviii] Food coloring, unless from natural food, should be avoided; it affects many children's health and behavior( )[xxix]. Health food stores have some tasty, naturally colored and sweetened Sundrops that look like M & M's.

The healthiest and best foods to eat are fresh (preferably organic) vegetables, fruits, grains, and nuts (unless allergic). Best meats are lean cuts, chicken, and fish. Again, free-range meats or meats with no chemical content are the healthiest. Most in our stores have been raised with hormones, antibiotics, and pesticide grains, but healthier choices are becoming more available. Check Pinterest, Facebook, and the PART II: FYI section in this book for healthy recipes.

Some of the healthiest people I know adhere to these basic foods. However, most of us find it difficult to cultivate this self-disciplined menu. When I first began changing foods and making healthier choices, I thought I would die! Ironically and conversely, the opposite happened; I didn't die but became healthier and healthier. Let's look at some healthier choices.

WHAT CHILDREN EAT

Meats

Meats should be limited. Now, that has been a hard one for this ole farm-raised girl! Since the body needs protein, choose other sources like beans, peas, nuts, and those listed in the PART II: FYI section.

If and when meat is eaten, choose fish, chicken, and turkey more often than pork or beef. Some professionals contend that beef and pork should be completely avoided. Choose fresh or frozen rather than processed, breaded, or canned meats. Try to get preservative/ chemical- free (no added hormones, antibiotics) meats. AVOID IRRADIATED MEATS! Watch the label *Natural*. Natural meat perhaps hasn't had chemicals added (a good thing) to it in processing, but were growth hormones, antibiotics, and other chemicals used in raising the live animals? Was the grain or food source loaded with chemicals?

Check your area to find growers of free-range chickens and turkeys. If you eat beef or pork, check for free-range or chemical-free animals. Also, ask your grocer about meats they have in stock or if they have access to healthier meats. These healthier choices cost more, so what I do is buy them but buy or consume less.

If lunch meats are necessary for your lifestyle, try brands like Boars Head that are minimally processed. Health food stores carry antibiotic /chemical-free meats.

Vegetables

"Yuk!" wail many children. "I don't like ve-guh-tuh-bles!" Because I observed my grandchildren's eating patterns, I believe this dislike to be caused by the enticing chemical additives in many fast- or- junk food products that have seduced their taste buds. They literally crave the unhealthy food and prefer it over the healthy. The healthier I eat and the longer I eat healthier foods, the less I desire junk food. When I do desire it and give in to that desire, my body often rejects it. My stomach or head hurts, I become congested or bloated, or I feel bad in general. Parents, PLEASE take a stand about vegetables for your children!

With veggies, buy fresh or frozen; raw is healthiest. Canned might be useful for occasional or emergency situations. As always, organic is best. It's especially important to buy organic carrots and other vegetables that are actually grown in the ground. (See PART II: FYI.) BEWARE of buying fresh vegetables in a store that has the detergent and air deodorizers anywhere near the open produce. Know that their toxins are going right into your food. Their VOC's can penetrate even bagged and boxed foods.

Fruits

Your child might not like fruit, especially if he or she has a "sweet tooth." Again, the chemical additives have affected the child's taste buds, training him to crave chemical sweets rather than natural. First, begin "weaning" from the processed sweets. Expect withdrawals and tantrums as the body cleanses from this sugar and white flour addiction. Immediately but gradually introduce fruits as replacements.

As with vegetables, fresh and frozen are good; organic is best. If there are no fresh, tasty fruits available, try frozen. READ THE LABELS to assure there are no sugars and other additives.

Real fruit is much healthier than juices, roll ups, and jellies. Fruit has pulp and fiber that the body needs; it converts to sugar more slowly. Also, it has fewer carbs and grams of sugar than artificial or extracted juices. (Note: Diabetes is epidemic in America. This disease directly correlates with diet, weight, and exercise. Help your child with both cancer and diabetes prevention.)

To emphasize again, if your child has had a diet high (even moderate) in sweets and carbs, he might have difficulty liking the taste of real fruits. It would be wise to keep unhealthy snacks out of your house. Stop for an occasional treat, but avoid bringing them into your house. Your children and you may have more self control than I have, but if junk food is in my house, it will eventually be eaten!

Breads/Grains/Nuts

Most breads and cereals on grocery shelves are unhealthy. They contain sugar (a lot of it, in some cases), high fructose corn syrup, preservatives, and other unhealthy chemicals. The benefits of whole wheat or whole grain are negated by the other undesirable contents.

After I became aware of the dangers of preservatives, I switched to a natural bread that had no preservatives, BUT it still contained sugar, dough conditioners, and other chemicals I could smell! (Imagine sniffing a piece of bread!) Now, I eat organic whole wheat or sprouted whole grain breads, still in limited amounts. Occasionally, I eat a burger or hot dog on a bun; again, <u>occasionally</u>.

Cereal is a popular breakfast food. Boxed or packaged cereals contain sugar as the first, second, or third ingredient— which means quite a bit of sugar. It may be necessary two to three days a week to use boxed cereal. If so, avoid food colors, high sugar, preservatives, or additives; READ THE LABELS. Try organic cereals, but even then, watch labels.

So, what about breakfast? Fruit is good for breakfast. A favorite breakfast of mine is toasted sprouted whole grain bread with either peanut or almond butter or a bit of butter and Simply Fruit (or similar) spread. Oatmeal is healthy and can be enhanced with fruit and/or nuts; it can be sweetened with honey, pure maple syrup, Stevia, or Xylitol…or pure cane or raw sugar. Free-range/organic scrambled or boiled eggs are good two or three times a week. Uncured(untreated) turkey bacon or bacon can be found. Healthy, modified muffins can be bought or made. (See recipes and resources in PART II: FYI.)

With breads and cereals, it is the processed white sugar and white flour to watch. And avoid additives and preservatives. Most of the hard-to-pronounce words are chemical additives.

<u>Desserts/Snacks</u>

This group tends to be the favorite of most children. Processed sugar and white flour are very tasty— and addictive. I've read that food additives create cravings, thus addictions, for consumers.[xxx] Notice: After eating sweets for a few days, a person might find an apple undesirable; however, after NOT eating sweets for a few days, a person would find that an apple actually tastes pretty good! If your child is to be healthier, snacks and desserts MUST be limited. Sugar lowers the immune system. Two to four sweets spread throughout the day causes the immune system to be impaired for the whole day. And don't forget about snacks that are carbs (chips, pasta, breads) for they will convert to sugar. Cancers feed on sugar. (See sugar list in PART II: FYI.)

If your child consumes snacks rather than healthy foods, he or she is not getting the nutrition needed to fight viruses and disease and to develop healthy tissues, organs, and bones. Desserts and snacks should be used after nutritious meals or sometimes between meals, NEVER in place of meals or before meals.

For desserts, try fresh or frozen fruits or fruit smoothies. Make homemade treats instead of having the boxed, packaged little cakes and cookies that are full of preservatives and other chemicals. We make pumpkin bread, oatmeal cookies, chocolate chip cookies, no bake cookies—all made with raw sugar or Xylitol, organic flour, and real butter or half amounts of vegetable oil. Annie's, Cascadian Farms, and Cliff make some delicious organic gummies and granola bars, flavored and colored with natural rather than artificial ingredients. Health food stores or organic sections in grocery stores provide many varieties of desserts and snacks.

Nuts are healthy snacks—UNLESS your child is allergic to them or is too young to consume them. Introduce these gradually and under a watchful eye. Tree nuts are especially healthy. Tasty nuts include pecans, almonds, cashews, macadamias, English and black walnuts, and pistachios. Sunflower and pumpkin seeds are healthy snacks as well.

Some possible snack ideas: (1) sliced banana with real peanut/almond butter and honey (2) sliced apple with cinnamon (Too tart? Add a bit of Stevia, Xylitol, honey, or pure maple syrup.) (3) berries-strawberries, blueberries, blackberries, raspberries (4) cinnamon toast (sprouted or wheat bread, real butter, cinnamon, and Xylitol/Stevia) (5) real fruit (6) fruit smoothies (7) favorite recipes modified (I love no-bake cookies and cobbler modified with Xylitol/Stevia, and whole wheat or gluten free flour).(See PART II: FYI.)

Most chips have no (or little) nutritional value and are often unhealthy. Of the many kinds with the long list of ingredients, choose one—-if you must have chips—with simple and few ingredients. I sometimes eat plain potato chips and Fritos; hardly ever do I eat the other flavorful chips for I think about the many chemicals that are in them. Know, too, that because chips are fried at high temps, the chemical *acrylamide* is produced. It is cancer causing and found highest in French fries and potato chips and other fried chips. My chip days have been ruined!!

AVOID sugar-free products!! Artificial sweeteners are chemicals that have been proven to have harmful side effects.[xxxi] Diabetic children may have to use sugar substitutes (so try Xylitol plus or Stevia to avoid the toxic chemicals), but a well-balanced diet of vegetables, whole grains and nuts, fruits, and lean meats might eliminate the need for use of sugar substitutes.

Look for helpful books and media information. READ LABELS! Make better choices. Your choices greatly determine the destiny of your child.

DRINKS CHILDREN CONSUME

What your child drinks is likewise very important to his health and well-being.

Water

Water is the essential drink.[xxxii] Without enough of it, a person can have many health complications. It carries sugar, nutrients, and hormones through the body, lubricates the joints, and aids in eliminating waste products. If dehydration occurs for lack of water, there are many health consequences.[xxxiii]Dehydration (lack of liquids) can lead to poor health, hospitalization, and even death if organs begin shutting down. Avoid water full of chemicals. Tap water is chlorinated, of course, and often heavily chlorinated; it sometimes tastes bad. Bottled waters can be a healthier choice, but some may not be as good as advertised. Testing has revealed chemicals in some. The main problem with bottled water is the plastic containers in which they are bottled. (Recommended documentary on Netflix: "Tapped") Spring and artesian waters are also better choices, if from a pure source. I had reverse osmosis installed on my tap water. One of my sisters boiled her tap water then put it through a Brita filter. Quality water has many benefits.

Juices

Juices may be very deceiving. Although the "healthy" juices do not contain all the chemicals of colas, many actually contain different additives and preservatives—and have high sugar content. Pure juice (100% fruit with no sugar added) is a better choice; still use these in moderation. Fresh or frozen whole fruit contain fiber and nutrients that are often missing in packaged or bottled juices. Caution: Avoid the colorful, popular fad drinks. They are full of color additives, dyes, chemicals, and sugars. READ THE CONTENT LABEL! This cannot be stressed enough.

Colas

Colas are an addictive mixture of chemicals—sugars, sugars, sugars, caffeine, preservatives, fillers. For health, NO CHILD SHOULD BE ALLOWED TO DRINK COLAS – especially the diet colas. Some parents allow daily or frequent consumption of colas! Not only is the child's immune system being shot (health), but also his behavior, mentality, and emotions are negatively affected.[xxxiv]

We wonder why our youth are having trouble with addictions(drug, alcohol, tobacco) and bad health (obesity, cancers, lethargy, viruses and cold, headaches, diabetes, ADHD, and behavior). Well, look around at all the drug conditioning to which our youth are being exposed—colas, candies and sweets, chips, fast foods. Junk foods contain multiple chemicals(drugs) that are habit forming, and the processing(especially of sugars) seems to contribute to the craving effect.[xxxv]

Tea & Coffee

It is well known that tea and coffee are stimulants that contain caffeine. Unless they are organic, they have been sprayed with chemicals. When I sit for hours in a coffee shop, I often walk out with a smell on my clothes, one that reminds me of cigarette smoke smell. Sometimes I awaken the next day with a sore throat or headache. My thoughts are, "Was this caused by the chemicals brewed off the coffee?"

An organic, naturally decaffeinated tea or coffee would be best, if your child is allowed to drink tea and coffee, but children will be affected by drinking tea and coffee that are stimulants.(FYI: Fibromyalgia recommendations include NO caffeine, sugar, and chemicals -fragrances included.)

CONCLUSION

We cannot totally avoid chemicals since we live in such a chemical world. Each parent, however, CAN make home safe (or safer) and collaborate with other parents and caregivers to make the child's school or daycare environment safer. Parents may contact companies and demand they quit making toxic products that are damaging, even killing, our children.

It is my prayer and hope that every child lover or child caretaker will apply the information in this book to their child's life. Please do it for the children. THINK AHEAD, years from now. Will the adult children in your family or care have healthy bodies, alert minds, acceptable behavior, and stable emotions? Will they be cancer free? Will they be assets or liabilities to society? Will they be thankful for the care you gave them or blame you for poor choices that damaged them for life?

1+1+1=3. SO, (1) DRINKING products that contain cancer-causing ingredients (carcinogens) + (2) EATING foods that contain cancer-causing ingredients (carcinogens) + (3) BREATHING chemicals and fragrances that contain cancer- causing ingredients(carcinogens) = possibility of CANCER—or other debilitating diseases.

What can YOU, as a child caregiver, do? (1) IDENTIFY foods and drinks you presently use that contain harmful chemicals, additives, and preservatives. (2) IDENTIFY the fragrant and chemical toxins your child breathes at home and at school. (3) GET RID OF THEM! MAKE HEALTHY CHANGES. Remember: One step at a time, but don't tarry. (4) CALL or WRITE companies that make your favorite products. Ask them to make healthy changes.

This is it in a nutshell. If you make healthy changes, your entire family will benefit. PLEASE, don't let your desires (to use unhealthy products) overcome your child's needs. If your family continues to eat, drink, and breathe toxic chemicals, THEY WILL SUFFER— now or in the future—especially the children. CHOOSE LIFE. Choose a healthier life. You CAN help keep your child from being 1 of the 36 (44 at last count) a Day…

THESE THINGS ARE HARD TO UNDERSTAND:

(1) Smokers who have children (especially those with ear infections, bronchitis, allergies, or asthma)— and they STILL smoke inside their homes and vehicles. Children with asthma, allergies, and ENT issues whose parents wear fragranced products and whose homes smell of candles, deodorizers, detergents, and other fragranced products.

(2) Schools, playgrounds, or sports fields that are next to busy highways with their toxic exhaust fumes or ones that have been built on or near landfills and other toxic waste areas or that are near industry that emits pollution.

(3) Avid sportsters who jog, bike, or walk on trails near busy highways and interstates. (Can't believe paths were constructed in these locations!) Their lungs are inhaling and their pores absorbing all that toxic exhaust!

(4) Stores with organic sections that are in close proximity to the detergent/air freshener sections. The once- organic products absorb fragrances and pesticides so, in reality, are no longer organic.

(5) Overweight people who constantly drink diet colas which contain additives that can make their cravings and weight problems escalate.

(6) People with cancer (or survivors), heart disease, diabetes, and other illnesses who still wear fragranced products and eat/drink chemical-laden

products. What a war their poor bodies wage! They not only have to fight the illnesses but also the toxins from the fragrances and chemicals. (I am this crazy-type person! I have diabetes and daily fight the battle with sweets and other carbs.)

(7) Health food store shoppers who are heavy fragrance users. The benefits they are deriving from their organic products are negated by their very inorganic, toxic fragrances.

(8) People who say they wear no fragrances yet smell very fragrant from their detergent, fabric softener, shampoo, hair gels, make-up, body soaps, or lotions. Fragrance is fragrance, no matter to which product it's been added. It still contains VOC's, pesticide, petroleum distillates, and many toxins which can be harmful to the respiratory, nervous, and reproductive systems— and contains one or more cancer-causing fillers.

(9) People with headaches, depression, or mood swings who wear fragrances   of any kind. This toxin goes right to work on their CNS, making them more depressed, escalating the head pounding, and causing their moods to swing even more, some almost to the point of bipolar symptoms.(I remember thinking I was perhaps bipolar. Praise God, I've had a chemical-free home for many years now, and I've not worried about that for a long time! AND I am in no way discounting bipolar illness.)

SIDENOTE TO CHRISTIANS AND CHURCHES

I am a Christian. I believe every word the Bible says. It says that Jesus came to give life. It also says that satan's* purpose and plan is to steal, destroy, or kill. His purpose from the beginning has been to destroy the seed of man— our children. His plan includes abuse, drugs and alcohol, accidents, and disease. From II Corinthians 1:4, *God* "who comforts us in all our troubles so that we can comfort those in any trouble with the comfort we ourselves have received from God,"[xxxvi] I believe that God allowed me to experience this long bout with chemical illness so that I might share with others what I learned: CHEMICALS ARE A TOXIC THREAT TO MANKIND. What more ironic way to harm our children than by the hands of the children's parents and teachers in their use of these chemicals in the home and school!

Nowhere (except at a perfume counter) do I smell more fragrances than at church. I am very concerned when I see a baby brought into a crowded service. Their little lungs and soft skin are exposed to myriad toxins from fragrances. At the beginning of services, I hear no one coughing; by the end, I often hear several coughing. Fragrances in church are as toxic as smoke in a lounge. One comes out covered with the smell of cigarettes or fragrances. The church's program, however, is God and His word. Sometimes I am so dizzy and dazed by the Sweet Poison that my mind cannot comprehend and grasp some of the sweet gospel.

KNOW that the fragrances most people are using are NOT the pure fragrance oils Mary poured over Jesus or the ones referenced in the Bible. Today's chemical fragrances are toxic and, in many cases, dangerous. Like many things made by the Lord for noble and good purposes (love, sex, music, food, money, fragrance), satan has added his poison and perverted their use.

Open your eyes; look around at the illnesses pervading our society. Quit burying your head in the sands of denial or self-indulgence. Logical deduction can surmise that satan is the driving force behind all the chemical toxicity in our country. God sure is NOT, for He is life, purity, and goodness. Isn't love of money—certainly not love of children—this driving force? The love of money is the root of (all kinds of) evil. Who is the father of lies, the lover of evil and death? I pray you quit listening to the Liar. Choose life and good health for your family.

*I will not capitalize the word satan.

MY STORY

I am not a physician, but I love people (especially children) and survived multiple chemical sensitivities (MCS or Environmental Illness). Allergies are not strangers to me. Since childhood mild allergies existed, but I was a strong, healthy person. Home cooked meals and hard work were constants in youth. Athletics brought me through junior and senior high schools. When the college lifestyle hit, my health declined somewhat. Processed foods, colas, and cigarettes entered. The junior high school habit of sleep deprivation, which grew with senior high, now intensified in college. My body's immune system was hard hit.

Careers of teaching and motherhood began. After 15 years of teaching, I developed more serious allergies. Eating habits improved and smoking stopped, but poor sleep habits remained. I blamed my few years of smoking for the bouts of bronchitis and sinus infections experienced. Because the school's janitorial cleaning products bothered me, I cleaned my own room at school, which added extra time and stress to an already busy day.

Over the years, my condition worsened. Fragrances irritated me, so I discontinued the use of perfumes and changed to mild musk. After a year or so, even that bothered me, as did fragrances of students and others. Many symptoms prevailed: headaches, depression, irritability, emotional meltdowns, sinus infections, breathing difficulty (asthma), bronchitis, and pneumonia. I thought I was going crazy and could hardly get out of bed, let alone teach a room full of teenagers. (Thankfully, my children were grown by this time.) I was sick or felt bad almost constantly.

After 23 years of teaching, my beloved profession came to an end. Since second grade, I wanted to be a teacher, so education had been a lifelong pursuit. I thought I would have to be "carried out of the classroom," which is what nearly happened— but for a different reason. I didn't reach retirement age; I had to quit because of illness. For almost eight years, I was virtually housebound and lived like a hermit. Depression and hopelessness overwhelmed me. NOT ONCE, in the first few years, DID I ASSOCIATE THIS ILLNESS WITH FRAGRANCES AND OTHER CHEMICALS.

Finally came the day of revelation! Three years into the debilitating illness, I ventured out of my house to an event. (I felt somewhat better since discontinuing the use of medications and beginning the use of natural supplements to cleanse and rebuild my body.) After a short time at the party, dizziness and fatigue hit me. A bit later, behavior and emotions changed; I needed to leave. The next day was one bleak continuum of depression and crying. Bronchitis struck. Another brain flick. Fragrances! I remembered smelling strong fragrances! My allergist had diagnosed multiple chemical sensitivities (more than allergies and asthma although similar), but I had never thought of fragrances as chemicals.

Years of research and prayer ensued. It is impossible to include in this book all I learned, but I have shared the basics. Time is short, and there is need for information NOW! This book is a place to begin. Then you can pursue your own quest and research about the toxins your family consumes.

Facts about additives, preservatives, and chemicals in what we eat, drink, and breathe point to cancer and other illnesses. I have personally experienced a few illnesses that I believe are directly related to these toxic products. All I know is that since I have cleaned my environment and changed my food/drink choices, I am much better.

Today, I am NOT housebound. I do not lead a normal life, but I am alive and well—until I get around too much fragrance and other toxins or eat foods loaded with preservatives and additives. I usually do NOT get a flu or virus many people have (as I once did). PRAISE GOD! My body is able to fight the germs since it isn't weary from continuous battle with chemicals. (v)

<table>
<tr><td align="center">ME</td><td align="center">ME</td></tr>
<tr><td align="center">⇩</td><td align="center">⇩</td></tr>
<tr><td align="center">Bacteria</td><td align="center">Bacteria</td></tr>
<tr><td align="center">Germs</td><td align="center">Germs</td></tr>
<tr><td align="center">Virus</td><td align="center">Chemical</td></tr>
<tr><td align="center"></td><td align="center">Chemical</td></tr>
<tr><td align="center"></td><td align="center">Chemical</td></tr>
<tr><td align="center"></td><td align="center">Virus</td></tr>
</table>

Get the picture? I can fight three things or an army.

There is no doubt in my mind or heart about the identity of the culprit (besides satan) that attacks and infests our children with cancer (and many other illnesses): CHEMICALS. WE HAVE BECOME A TOXIC, CHEMICAL SOCIETY! Unless the home and/or school are fragrance and chemical free, children eat, drink, and breathe harmful toxins 24 hours a day. This is tragic! And our dear children are paying the price! Know that fragrances (unless essential oils) are among the most deceiving in the environmental world, thus the name SWEET POISON.

Fragrances are used everywhere and are in most personal care and household cleaning products. EWG (Environmental Working Group) states that, "…top-selling fragrance products…contain a dozen or more secret chemicals not listed on labels, multiple chemicals that can trigger allergic reactions or disrupt hormones…"[xxxvii] The President's Cancer Panel sounded an alarm over the understudied and largely unregulated toxins used by millions of Americans in their daily lives. Hormone disruptors that play a role in cancer were found in many of the fragrances analyzed for this study.[xxxviii] Nova Scotia (Canada) Allergy and Environmental Health Assoc. did an extensive two-year study about the dangers of household chemicals and fragrances.[xxxix] In the fall of 2009, the CDC (Center for Disease Control and Prevention) composed a multi-page policy about fragrances. They have required their facilities be as FRAGRANCE-FREE as possible.[xl] They are to be applauded. CDC studies disease control, so what does this tell us? Obvious!

It is my hope and prayer that every parent, grandparent, teacher, and daycare provider read this book. As previously stated, *36 A DAY!* is not an all-inclusive resource with complete information. It is, however, a place for you to begin making your child's environment a safer, healthier one in which he or she may flourish, not wilt. Perhaps your precious child will be spared a journey of illness.

If you truly value the children in your life, you WILL do something— or at least try—to keep them from becoming 1 of the 36 a day (actually, 44 a day in 2015) diagnosed with cancer. I appeal to most of you parents and caregivers who DO care much. Some will not have any desire to read this book and face its issues; they deny problems and "hide their heads in the sand." Others, sadly, do not care enough or care more for themselves and their wants rather than their children's needs. Still others will read the book but ignore its contents and warnings. (They don't realize that cancer and illness do not happen overnight; illness is usually a few years in the developmental stage.) And some will read but rationalize that their drug of choice, Sweet Poison, has no effect on their children. Hmmm, SWEET POISON. Thank God, however, many will choose life and health for their children and will take action immediately! They will give their children an opportunity to grow up—and grow old.

In Part II: FYI (For Your Information) are several resources for your use. However, I encourage you to do your own research. In this book, I shared basic information about healthier food, drink, and air for your family. This information, if you act on it, could keep your beloved child from being 1 of 36 diagnosed with cancer—tomorrow, next week, next month, next year. It could even help you!

I must be as factual and straightforward as possible. I apologize now to any fragrance lovers who are offended and don't want to give up your scents. My concern is FOR THE CHILDREN.

(Problem Solver: Switch from toxic chemical fragrances to pure essential oil fragrances!!)

PART II: FOR YOUR INFORMATION (FYI)

In this section is much helpful information. It includes DEFINITIONS of terms or concepts with which you might not be familiar; RESOURCES to which you can refer for answers to questions you might have; FURTHER READING of related articles for those who want to do more research; DANA'S CORNER, a Colorado friend's personal comments and recipes; RECIPES/ ALTERNATIVES to chemical products; NOTEWORTHY ADDITIONAL INFORMATION; and SUMMARIES of articles related to this book's subject (toxic chemicals and cancer) plus extras.

It is impossible to tell you all I've learned and lived in my 20 years of research and experience. I have boxes and stacks of documentation and information about the dangers of chemicals. Chemicals—especially fragrances—were the cause of a debilitating illness which ended my teaching profession of almost 25 years and caused about 15 years of health issues, eight of which were spent mostly in isolation. Hopefully, what is shared in this book and its reference section will help you have a healthier home (thus family) and make more informed choices. Remember: PLEASE do your own research!

DEFINITIONS

Ataxia-loss of muscle coordination

Carcinogen-cancer producing substance

CEHN-Children's Environmental Health Network; a national multidisciplinary project whose purpose is to protect the health of children as it relates to environmental hazards

CDC-Center for Disease Control and Prevention

CIIN-Chemical Injury Information Network

CNS-Central Nervous System (brain and spine)

CNS Disorders-dementia, MS(multiple sclerosis), Parkinson's, Alzheimer's, seizures, strokes, SIDS(sudden infant death syndrome),ADD(attention deficit disorder)

EPA-Environmental Protection Agency

EWG-Environmental Working Group (highly rated)

FDA- Federal Food and Drug Administration

Formaldehyde-colorless, pungent irritating gas used chiefly as a disinfectant and a preservative; used…fertilizers, dyes, and embalming fluids (*Merriam Webster)*

Free Radicals-molecule capable of multiplying rapidly and harming the immune system

H.E.A.L.-Human Ecology Action League

Irradiated Meats and Foods-Irradiation is the process of using carefully controlled amounts of ionizing radiation on food to help eliminate disease-causing microorganisms like

E. coli and salmonella, parasites, mold, and bacteria. It is used to prolong shelf life of fruits and vegetables as it inhibits sprouting and delays ripening. It also sterilizes. The FDA has approved irradiation of meat and poultry and allows its use for other foods.

MSDS-Material Safety Data Sheet (ingredients/contents list)

Organic-of produce grown without pesticides; of living organisms

Paraben-chemical preservative that mimics estrogen in our bodies which can be absorbed through skin or inhaled

Phthalates-plasticizers; group of chemicals used to make plastics more flexible and hard to break (CDC)

Protein Sources-Proteins are all foods made from meat, poultry, seafood, beans and peas, eggs, nuts, and seeds. (protein.com) Health.com lists the best vegan and vegetarian protein sources. Proteins are the building blocks of life and promote cell growth and repair. Animal proteins can be high in saturated fats and cholesterol. Fourteen good vegan sources include green peas, quinoa, nuts and nut butter (with as few ingredients as possible), beans, chickpeas, tempeh and tofu, edamame, leafy greens, hemp seeds, chia seeds, seeds, seitan, non-dairy milk, and unsweet cocoa powder. (Women need 46 grams, men 56 grams of protein daily.)

Sensitizer-damaging to the immune system

<u>VOC's</u>-volatile organic compounds; ones that evaporate rapidly; explosive; ones that cannot be contained, thus spreading throughout an area

RESOURCES-GUIDES

This section is, by no means, all-inclusive. These are merely a few resources to give you additional information. These five (5) resources were invaluable to me on my journey to wellness. Most can be found online.

(1) *The Human Ecologist*-publication from Human Ecology Action League (H.E.A.L.); back issues available

(2) *Our Toxic Times*-publication from Chemical Injury Information Network (CIIN) that features several articles about cancer, as well as many other health issues; back issues available

(3) www.anapsid.org -list of recommended personal care products (deodorant, shampoo & conditioner, hair gel, hand & body soap, body & moisturizing lotion, sunscreen, shaving cream, lipstick, laundry, etc.)

(4) www.hallgold.com – Toxic Chemical Ingredients (cosmetics and body care products)- a very comprehensive ingredient directory based upon MSDS (material safety data sheets)information

(5) www.lesstoxicguide.ca –The Guide to Less Toxic Products (Nova Scotia Allergy & Environmental Health Association.) People are increasingly aware that many products contain ingredients that pose serious risks to human health, but they often don't know where to start to find less toxic products. The Guide was developed to make it easier to make healthy choices. Says project coordinator Barb

Harris,"…the most effective way to deal with illness is to prevent it." This VERY informative study was a two-year study. Hundreds of brand names were evaluated, as well as toxic ingredients used in cosmetics and personal care items, household cleaners, and baby care products. (Also included are some homemade household cleaner recipes.)

RESOURCES – GROUPS

American College of Preventive Medicine (www.acpm.org) – physicians dedicated to preventing known potential routes of exposure to environmental hazards (ingestion, absorption, inhalation); children's susceptibility to environmental hazards; one of the nation's leading pediatric environmental health experts

American Association for Cancer Research – oldest and largest professional association related to cancer research

Alternative Medicine.com

American Cancer Society

Beyond Pesticides- national coalition against misuse of pesticides

CEHN (Children's Environmental Health Network) – national multidisciplinary project whose purpose is to protect the health of children as it relates to environmental hazards (www.cehn.org)

Coalition for Healthier Schools (518-462-0632)

Consumer Product Safety Commission

CDC National Center for Environmental Health

Environmental Health Coalition

Fragranced Products Information Network

Friends of the Earth – engages in bold, justice-minded environmentalism; 45 year history (www.foe.org)

Green School- a Nationwide Environmental Learning Program (Project Learning Tree) greenschools.org)

Healthy Schools Network, Inc. (www.healthyschools.org) - 1995; a leading voice for children's environmental health at school

Healthy Schools – Massachusetts Public Health Association, "Healthy Kids: The Keys to Basics"

Improving Kids' Environments (ikecoalition.org)

National Children's Cancer Society

National (and local) PTA

National Institute for Health (NIH) –U.S. Dept. of Health; one of the world's foremost medical research centers; national center for environmental health

National Institute of Environmental Health Sciences (list of common indoor air pollutants)

Robbins Environmental Medicine Center (1985), Dr. Albert Robbins, Boca Raton, FL

Right-to-Know Network

Sierra Club

St. Jude Children's Research Hospital – Memphis, TN; ranked one of the best pediatric cancer hospitals in the country; first and only national cancer institute designated a comprehensive cancer center devoted solely to children

Truth in Labeling Campaign

Women's Environmental Network (1992) – fosters professional networks for women working to protect the environment

World Health Organization (WHO) – addresses children's environmental health risks

RESOURCES – BOOKS

- Col. Joe Hart. *Cancer Cure.*
- Gerson, Charlotte and Morton Walker, D.P.M. *The Gerson Therapy :The Proven Nutritional Program for Cancer and Other Illnesses.* New York: Kensington Publishing Corp., 2006.
- Gerson, Dr. Max. *The Gerson Miracle: A Cancer Therapy Book.*
- Gilbere, Dr. Gloria. *Chemical Cuisine: Do You Really Know What You're Eating?* (www.gloriagilbere.com)
- Hubbard, Dr. Ron. *Clear Body, Clear Mind: The Effective Purification Program.* 2002. www.clearbodyclearmind.com. (all natural program to eliminate accumulated drugs and toxins in the body and mind)New York Times Bestseller.
- Kosta, Louise A. *Fragrance and Health.* Atlanta, GA: Human Ecology Action League, 1998.
- *International Journal of Oncology.* (international journal dedicated to oncology research and cancer treatment).
- Zukowski, Shea. *All-You-Need All-Stars of the Home.* (salt, lemons, vinegar, and baking soda) Amazon.

RESOURCES – DOCUMENTARIES

*Netflix has available some of these documentaries. There are many informative ones online.

Food, INC

Forks over Knives

Tapped (water and plastic)

Food Matters

Super Size Me

Gerson Therapy

FURTHER READING
FRAGRANCES

*Almost all of these articles may be found online in the form entered here. I had to alter the bibliographic order of some so they would be more easily accessed.

"The Addictive Power of Toxic Perfumes and Colognes." June 18, 2011. www.Healthimpactnews.com.

Anderson, Ava. "Five 'Must-Knows' on the Dangers of Synthetic Fragrance." *Health, Health and Fitness, Organic Living,* Feb. 6, 2014 (natural beauty expert and safe cosmetics advocate). www.mariasfarmcountrykitchen.com.

Booth, Barbara. "Perfume, Perfume Everywhere." Environmental Science and Technology online, June 1, 2007. www.researchgate.net/6225946.

Bridges, Betty, RN. "Fragrance: Emerging Health and Environmental Concerns." Oct. 2002. John Wiley and Sons, Vol. 17, Issue 5. DOI: 10.10021ffj.1106. www.onlinelibrary.wiley.com.

CDC-"Indoor Environmental Quality." Chemicals-odors. Nov. 3, 2015. www.cdc.gov/.

"Chemical Risk to Future Fertility." British Broadcasting Corp. News. Aug. 31, 2008. news.bbc.co.uk.

"College Campus without Scents?" *Modesto Bee.* www.modbee.com/news/local.

DesJardins, Andrea. "Sweet Poison: What Your Nose Can't Tell You about the Dangers of Perfume." Health and Environmental Resource Center, 1977. www.jrussellshealth.org.

Franz, Damon and Holly Prall. "Smelling Good but Feeling Bad." Toxics Information Project, *Green Living* e-magazine. www.toxicsinfor.org/personal.

The Herald Sun News. "Terror Strike – London."(killer used posh perfume in bombs) London, July 7, 2005. www.freerepublic.com/focus/news.

King, Elisabeth. "Growing Argument for a Fragrance-Free Environment." adapted from *The Age*. Australia, July 2004. www.ciin.org/news.

Kosta, Louise. "Speaking Up about Environmental Fragrance." *The Human Ecologist,* winter 2007.

"Perfume Aromas Prove Costly to Detroit in ADA Settlement." March 17, 2010. www.insidecounsel.com.

Pitts, Connie. "One Woman's Perfume—Another Woman's Poison." *Let's Live,* 2003. (invisible chemical poisons)

Potera, C. Indoor Air Quality: "Scented Products Emit a Bouquet of VOC's." National Center for Biotechnology Information, *Environmental Health Perspectives,* Jan. 2011. (A single fragrance in a product can contain a mixture of hundreds of chemicals.) www.ncbi.nlm.nih.gov.

Sarantis, Heather, MS; Olgev Naidenko, PhD; Sean Gray, MS; Jane Houlihan, MSE; and Stacy Malkan. "Not-so-Sexy: The Health Risks of Secret Chemicals in Fragrances."

Campaign for Safe Cosmetics and EWG, May 2010. www.ewg.org.

"Scented Consumer Products Shown to Emit Many Unlisted Chemicals." *Science News*, Oct. 26, 2010. www.sciencedaily.com/releases.

Sherman, Amy (posted). "What Stinks at BSO's Internal Affairs Office?" (fragrances banned at sheriff's office) *The Miami Herald,* May 12, 2010. miamiherald.typepad.com/.

"Smells Make Some People Sick." *Science Daily,* Jan. 2, 2012. www. sciencedaily.com.

Steinemann, Anne C., PhD. (civil and environmental engineer) and colleagues. "Even 'Green' Scented Products May Emit Hazardous Chemicals." *Environmental Impact Assessment Review*, University of Washington, Feb. 11, 2013. News.discovery.com/human.

Thomas, John D. and Brian Shilhavy. "Is Your Health Being Destroyed by Toxic Fragrances?" *Health and Fitness,* 2014. https://books.google.com/books.

LAUNDRY

Cutler, Nicole, L.AC. "Fabric Softeners and Your Liver." Aug. 12, 2011. www.liversupport.com.

Hickey, Hannah. "Scented Laundry Products Emit Hazardous Chemicals." University of Washington, Aug. 24, 2011. www.washington-edu/.

Kessler, Rebecca. "Dryer Vents: An Overlooked Source of Pollution." *Environmental Health Perspective,* Nov. 1, 2011. Ehp.niehs.nih.gov/119-a474a.

Louis, PF. "Beware of Hidden Toxin Sources in New Clothes." *International Business Times*, Sept. 3, 2012. www.naturalnews.com,1037038.

Moran, Barbara. "EPA Investigating Toxic Laundry Emissions in New England." *The Hartford Courant,* Nov. 20, 2012. Articles.courant.com/.

Spencer, Ben (science reporter). "Doctor's Orders: Why You Should Always Wash New Clothes." (chemicals, insects – Prof. Donald Belsito, dermatologist, Columbia University Medical Centre)*The Daily Mail,* May 20, 2015. www.dailymail.co.uk/.

AIR FRESHENERS/DEODORIZERS

"Air Fresheners or Air Poisoners?" Seeds for Change Wellness. seedsforchangewellness.com.

BBC News. "Air Fresheners and Aerosols Harm Mothers and Children." Oct. 19, 2004. News.bbc.co.uk 3752188.

"Chemical Air Fresheners Harm Your Indoor Air Health." Mar. 19, 2014. www.sylvane.com.

"Glade Air Freshener: Poster Child for Toxic Secrets." May 20, 2013. https://www.momsrising.org.

Hickman, Martin. "Breast Cancer Link to Cleaning Products and Air Fresheners." Health News, *The Independent,* July 20, 2010. www.independent.co.uk.

Kay, Jane (environmental writer). "Environmental Groups Petition U.S. to Regulate Air Fresheners." adapted from *San Francisco Chronicle,* Sept. 20, 2007. www.sfgate.com.

"New Study Finds Scented Candles and Air Fresheners Pose Dangerous Health Risks." Dec. 18, 2015. www.womansday.com/health.

Peplow, Mark. "Fears Raised as Plug-ins Linked to Cancer Compounds," ("Air Fresheners Cause a Stink.") May 10, 2004. www.nature.com/news 040503.

"Teen Dies from Inhaling Air Freshener." Associated Press, April 14, 2005. (several incidents of this)

PERSONAL CARE

"Antibacterial Soap Is No More Effective than Regular Soap." *Forbes,* Sept. 28, 2015. www.forbes.com

"Body Absorbs 5 Pounds of Make-up a Year." April 23, 2015. thoughtcatalog.com.

"Dangerous Beauty: 5 Scariest Beauty Products." *Forbes,* March 12, 2012. www.forbes.com.

"Environmental Exposure to Hairspray, Lipstick, and Pollution Can Trigger Autoimmune Diseases." Organic Consumers Association, Feb. 11, 2010. https://www.organicconsumers.

"Plain Soap as Effective as Antibacterial Soap without the Risk." *Science Daily,* Aug. 16, 2007. (many related articles)

"Popular Shampoos Contain Toxic Chemicals Linked to Nerve Damage." Jan. 11, 2005. www.naturalnews.com/003210.

Stokes, Paul. "Body Absorbs 5 lbs. of Make-up Chemicals a Year." Telegraph Media Group, Ltd., *UK News,* June 22, 2007. www.telegraph.co.uk.

Sohn, Emily. "Baby Products Loaded with Toxins." *Discovery News,* May 18, 2011. News.discovery.com/human.

"Toxic Beauty Ingredients to Avoid." *Huffington Post,* Nov. 12, 2013. www.huffingtonpost.com/.

"Toxic Chemicals in Kids' Bath Products." EWG, March 12, 2009. www.ewg.org/.

CLEANERS

"CleanYour House without the Toxins." Dr. Frank Lipman. Feb. 7, 2013. www.drfranklipman.com.

Greensfelder, Liese. "Study Warns of Cleaning Product Risk." University of CA- Berkeley, May 22, 2006. berkeley.edu/.

Guide to Healthy Cleaning. EWG. Breakdown of numerous cleaning products into A, B, C, D, and F ratings.

Guide to Less Toxic Products. Nova Scotia Allergy and Environmental Health Assoc. (two-year study with many categories) *Excellent, extensive!

"Hidden Hazards Found in Green Products." University of Melbourne press release, March 5, 2015. Themelbourneengineer.eng.unimelb.edu.

Van Noppen, Donnell (Trip). "Getting the Dirt on Household Cleaners." Earthjustice; adapted from commentary for *Earthjustice,* Feb. 17, 2010. Earthjustice.org/blog.

"Your Cleaning Products Might Be More Harmful than You Think." www.realsimple.com

PESTICIDES

*Note: Pesticides are in many cleaning products—even fragrances— not only in insecticides.

Beyond Pesticides. April 22, 2004. (current actions and newsletters including pesticide safety) www.beyondpesticides.org.

"Insect Repellent DEET Linked to Penis Defects (Hypospadias)." News.com.au, Dec. 1, 2009. www.news.com.au.

"Pesticides Tied to Childhood Cancers." *New York Times,* Sept. 21, 2005. Well.blogs.nytimes.com.

"Pesticide Use at Home Linked to Childhood Cancer Risk." CBS News, Sept. 14, 2015. www.cbsnews.com/.

Rundant, Jeremie, et al. "Pesticide Exposure and Higher Risk of Childhood Cancers." *Environmental Health Perspectives,* Sept. 25, 2007.

Shaply, Dan. Study: "Home Pesticides Linked to Childhood Cancer, The Daily Green." *Seattle Post – Intelligencer,* Aug. 29, 2010.

"Study Links Childhood Cancer and In-Home Pesticide Use." EWG, Sept. 28, 2015. www.ewg.org.

"Study of Pesticides and Children Stirs Protests." *The Washington Post,* Oct. 30, 2004. (EPA and chemical industry want to pay families to expose children to pesticides, two times a month for two years, so 48 exposures!)( ) (My note: unbelievable and inhuman! In America?!) www.washingtonpost.com.

FOOD

"Dump Your Doritos, Fritos, and Cheetos! There's No Excuse for Eating Junk Food." *The Huffington Post.* May 24, 2014. www.huffingtonpost.com

"Food Additives to Avoid." EWG. www.ewg.org.

"Healthy Snacks to Replace Chips." Sara Ipatenco. Feb. 18, 2014. www.livestrong.com>Food & Drink

Kobylewski, Sarah, PhD. Candidate, and C. Michael Jacobsen, Executive Director CSPI. "Food Dyes: A Rainbow of Risks." News release from Center for Science in the Public Interest, June 29, 2010. https://cspinet.org/

Meeker, Susan and Larry & Jennifer Ferrare. "Meat Monopolies: Dirty Meat and the False Promises of Irradiation." Food and Water Report.

"Pediatricians Say Flamin' Hot Cheetos Are Burning Your Kids' Insides." Nov. 19, 2013. Jezebel.com/pediatricians

"Potato Chip Warnings." Sara Ipatenco. Jan. 28, 2015. Livestrong.com.

Sagon, Candy. "Eight Foods We Eat That Other Countries Ban." AARP, June 25, 2013. blog.aarp.org.

CANCER

"Are We Bathing Our Babies in Carcinogens?" Campaign for Safe Cosmetics Study. Douglass Report, April 1, 2009. (CSC found products like Johnson & Johnson baby shampoo contained chemicals the EPA has marked as probable carcinogens.)

"Better Than Chemo: Turmeric Kills Cancer Not Patients." Sept. 17, 2015. the internetpost.net.

"Cancer Health Risk Significantly Underestimated by EPA (VOC's)." Bloomberg School of Public Health. March 3, 2004. (also John Hopkins University) www.sciencedaily.com/releases040303075116.

CDC. "Higher Cancer Risk for Kids Living Near Busy Roads." *USA Today,* March 20, 2014. www.usatoday.com/story.

Gucciardi, Anthony. "Study Accidentally Finds Chemotherapy Makes Cancer Far Worse." Natural Society, Aug. 7, 2012. naturalsociety.com.

"Johnson & Johnson Promises to Remove Carcinogens from Baby Products." PR Newswire, U.S. Newswire, and Women's Voices for the Earth, Nov. 17, 2011. www.prnewswire.com/. (My note and concern: Why were the CARCINOGENS in our baby products in the first place?? An outrage!!)

"Rise in Childhood Cancers Parallels Toxic Chemical Proliferation." Environmental News Service, Jan. 26, 2011. www.ens-newswire.com.

The Truth about Cancer: A Global Quest. A nine- episode documentary series, Dec. 23, 2015. www.naturalnews.com. (I have seen only a bit of this; it's recommended by one of the sites I read.)

Warburg, Prof. O. "On the Origin of Cancer Cells." National Center for Biotechnology Information, *Science,* 1956. DOI: 10.1126.

GENERAL

"Air Pollution Deaths on the Rise…" CNN.com, Sept. 16, 2015. www.cnn.com.

American Lung Association. "600 Ingredients in Cigarettes." www.lung.org.

"Are Cells the New Cigarettes?" *New York Times,* June 26, 2010. www.nytimes.com.

"Cell Phones: The New Cigarettes?" *Scientific American,* Ronald Herberman. www.scientificamerican.com.

"Chemicals in Tobacco Smoke." Center for Disease Control & Prevention (CDC). Mar. 21, 2011. www.cdc.gov/tobacco (A mix of 7,000+ chemicals, hundreds of which are toxic; 70 cause cancer).

Choosing Safer Products: Art & Craft Supplies. watoxics.org/files/art hobby.

"Consequences of Lack of Water." Sylvia Tremblay, MSc. June 10, 2015.

Clementine Art Supplies. (all natural art supplies)

"Creativity without Chemicals." Washington Toxics Coalition, Sept. 2011. www.watoxics.org.

Grossman, Elizabeth. "Untested Chemicals Are Everywhere, Thanks to Obsolete TSCA (Toxic Substance Control Act)." *The Guardian,* Feb. 13, 2015. www.theguardian.com.

Janssen, Dr. Sarah. "Toxic Chemicals in Pregnant Women." Feb. 7, 2011. simplesteps.org.

Ketcham, Christopher. "Warning: Your Cell Phone May Be Hazardous to Your Health." *GQ,* Jan. 25, 2010. www.gq.com.story.

"Lack of Drinking Water Deteriorates Human Body." April 16, 2015. www.medicaldaily.com

"Landmark Scientific Statement on Early Chemical Exposure and Lifelong Health." International Conference of Experts on Environmental Health, Environmental Chemistry, Developmental Biology, Toxicology, Epidemiology, Nutrition, and Pediatrics. May, 2007.

Layton, Lyndsey. "Use of Potentially Harmful Chemicals Kept Secret under Law." *Washington Post,* Jan. 4, 2010. www.washingtonpost.com.

Mercola, Dr. Joseph. "10 Things to Throw Away for Better Health." April 6, 2015. World's #1 natural health website. articles.mercola.com.

"Pollution May Cause 40% of Global Deaths." Sept. 10, 2007. www.livescience.com.

Rust, Susanne and Meg Kissinger. "EPA Puts Children at Risk by Dropping the Ball on Chemical Dangers." *Milwaukee Journal Sentinel,* March 30, 2008. www.jsonline.com.

Shapley, Dan. (30) "New Toxic Chemicals to Avoid." June 17, 2009. thedailygreen.com.

WHO: "7 Million Premature Deaths Annually Linked to Air Pollution." World Health Organization, March 25, 2014. www.who.int/mediacentre.

WHO: "30% of Diseases in Children Result from the Environment." World Health Organization. (preventing disease through healthy environments). www.who.int/...preventingdisease.

Young, Saundra. "Researchers List Chemicals Endangering the Next Generation of Brains." CNN, Feb. 17, 2014. www.cnn.com.

DANA'S CORNER
BIO

"I'm Dana Abrahamson, and I'm blessed to live in the Colorado mountains in a small, historic town called Georgetown. With my husband Craig, I have two teenage daughters and an elementary age son. (I met my friend and the author of this book, Judy Dees, because she purchased some land, and I'm a realtor.) Over the last several years, I've come to some conclusions: I don't want to expose my family to harmful chemicals and pesticides; I don't want to squander my family's resources on things we simply don't need; and I want to know that I have the skills to be self-sufficient to the greatest possible degree. To me, this means using basic, inert ingredients to make as many products as we need to keep a clean home, wash our clothes and dishes, and take good care of our health and personal needs.

I didn't learn how to garden or cook overnight, and I certainly didn't start using natural products with my own recipes all at once. It's a gradual process and should be enjoyable to you. If you have no interest in soap-making, there are some nice options for purchase that aren't filled with fragrance, parabens, and surfactants. There are skills and levels of knowledge and sophistication that you will gain over time.

I think a great place to start is laundry…the recipes are simple, affordable, and will work with any machine in any place. The positive impacts on your family and the environment are immeasurable. Best of all, your clothes will be clean! More difficult is hair care, but try some of the ideas here and experiment until you find what works for you. It really is worth it, and just think of the money you won't spend and the plastic bottles you won't add to the world. Even if you recycle, it's a much better option to choose not to consume in the first place. And try not to be intimidated by what seems like a time-consuming endeavor.

Most of us don't have the luxury of full-time homemaking, and yet we can simplify our lives and make better decisions for our families in less time and with less money than you ever imagined. Start where you are and go at the pace you want. Don't doubt yourself or worry about making a mistake. Ignore people who wouldn't dream of using homemade deodorant and know that these choices are so much better. Soon you'll be handing out homemade deodorant recipes with abandon!

My kids and their friends like to laugh about how 'weird' I am. In their lunches, they have glass and stainless steel containers of things like homemade yogurt, organic fruit, and grass-fed beef. My more sun-sensitive daughter will not use my homemade sun block, and the athlete refuses to use homemade deodorant. My son cannot choke down homemade elderberry syrup for a cold. But I know they're learning to make good choices every day, and I know they secretly don't even think I'm that weird. I know they are strong and healthy, and I feel good that I don't expose them to things that will hurt them today or fifty years from now.

And the journey continues."

(My note: Dana, I'm so proud of you for making the decision to go healthy. Yes, years down the road is when your children, Craig, and you will know the difference. Thank you much for sharing what you are learning. I bet you thought I was 'weird' when we started talking about all this several years ago! Glad you are 'on board,' Healthy Momma!)

DANA'S NOTES

Great snacks include smoothies; raw veggie juice; apples, peanut butter, <u>dark</u> chocolate chips; bananas, honey, and peanut butter. Lemon water is a refreshing drink.

Because many of the ingredients I use are on amazon.com, I have $100 yearly membership to Amazon Prime. Benefits include free two-day shipping, lots of digital content like music and books, and good products.

www.WellnessMomma.com. is another good website. They have many items including the homemade deodorant, sunscreen, elderberry syrup, Vitamin D3, probiotics, Omega 3, and other supplements and health items. See Kim's Corner for essential oil diffuser recipes.

I use apple cider vinegar and honey for general good health. (My note: I use oregano oil and elderberry juice for general good health. I think I will try Dana's for it's much less expensive and has been in use for years.) Diabetics might find sw cactus, bilberry, and cinnamon helpful.

I use essential oils rather than chemical fragrances. Most health food stores sell diffusers; they are found online, too. Simply add water and a healthy fragrant essential oil of choice and your house smells great WITHOUT the danger of toxic chemical fragrances.

RECIPES

<u>Laundry</u>

Detergent: (Most ingredients may be found in the laundry section of stores.)

Borax	4 lb. 12 oz. box
Washing Soda	3 lb. 7 oz. box
Baking Soda	4 lb. box
Oxyclean	3 lb. box (get the *Free* type, not ones with blue crystals)

Mix in a big tub; then put in smaller containers. Use 1 Tbs. in laundry (2 Tbs. if dirty) and sprinkle on top of clothes. I like to add 1 Tbs. Dr. Bronner's Sal Suds (health food stores) in the detergent dispenser.

Fabric Softener: In a gallon jug, add 2 cups white vinegar and fill with warm water. (You may also add a few drops of pure essential oils, found at health food stores. I like peppermint, bergamot, etc. Cedarwood or tea tree are good antibacterials.) Add ½ cup of mix to each load in softener dispenser. In the dryer, put nothing.

Personal Care

Hair Wash: Boil 2+ cups water. In a container, mix 1 ½ cups of the water and 2 Tbs. baking soda. (This is enough for 4-6 applications). With shampoo (which causes your hair to over produce oil, thus necessitates daily washing), we are used to lots of suds. Hardly any suds here! Pour into an applicator or old shampoo bottle. Wet your hair, then squirt mix on hair line and rub it in. It runs down the hair shafts. Rinse hair well before putting on vinegar rinse.

Hair Rinse: You may want to rinse hair with straight white vinegar for a month or so to get off old residue. (Some people use pure soap to clean hair, but a film is left on the hair; it won't rinse out in hard water.) OR you may dilute white vinegar, 1 Tbs. in ½ cup warm water then pour over hair. Don't rinse (Vinegar smell dissipates quickly and isn't toxic.). Vinegar is acidic and will close hair follicles and will smooth and soften. Some people use apple cider vinegar, but it makes my hair limp and oily. It might work for you, if you have coarse, dry hair. If you desire milder, try lemon juice instead. Try rinsing and not rinsing to see which your hair needs. Curly hair? Google co-wash.com, a conditioning wash one of my daughters uses sometimes. Amazon has a coconut mango co-wash. Also available is the co-wash As I Am.

Toothpaste: Mix the following: 1 Tbs. baking soda, 1 Tbs. sea salt, and bentonite clay. For flavor, add dry mint leaves, cloves, cinnamon, or your favorite essential oil. Another: Mix 4 Tbs. bentonite clay, 3 Tbs. calcium magnesium powder, 1 Tbs. baking soda, 2 Tbs. powdered mint or a few drops mint essential oil or another flavor, 1 Tbs. cinnamon, 1 tsp. clove powder, 1 Tbs. Xylitol, essential oil for taste.

Sunscreen: Combine all the following ingredients <u>except</u> zinc oxide. Warm the ingredients in a water bath. Stir in zinc oxide. Pour into a container and cool. Ingredients: ½ cup almond or olive oil; ¼ cup coconut oil (natural spf 4); ¼ cup beeswax; 2 Tbs. shea butter; 2 Tbs. zinc oxide (non-nano). Optional: 1 tsp. Vitamin E oil. Optional: essential oil, vanilla extract.

<u>Foods</u>

Coffee Creamer: In a blender, mix 19 oz. can coconut milk, 2 Tbs. unrefined coconut oil, 1 tsp. vanilla, and 2 Tbs. unsulphured black strap molasses (I like Plantation brand). Blend all and put in a quart mason jar. Refrigerate.

Chocolate Cinnamon Bread (for bread machine):

Small Loaf (1 lb)	Ingredients	Large Loaf (1 ½ lb.)
¾ cup + 2 Tbs.	hot brewed coffee	1 ¼ cup
¼ cup	unsweet cocoa powder	1/3 cup
1 ½ tsp.	active dry yeast	2 ¼ tsp.
1 ¾ cup	bread flour	2 2/3 cups
1/3 cup	whole wheat flour	½ cup
2 Tbs.	sugar,(Xylitol, Stevia)	3 Tbs.
½ tsp.	salt	¾ tsp.
1 tsp.	ground cinnamon	1 ½ tsp.
2 Tbs.	veggie oil	3 Tbs.

Pour hot coffee into a small bowl. Add the cocoa and stir till dissolved and smooth. Let cool to room temp.

Add all ingredients in the order suggested by your bread machine manual and process on the bread cycle according to manufacturer's directions. (I have this ready in the morning for my kids.)

<u>Miscellaneous</u>

Cider Vinegar: In a 2 qt. pitcher, add almost 2 qt. cold water, ¼ cup raw honey, and ¼ cup apple cider vinegar (Braggs brand w/Mother). Mix well. Serve over ice. This is good for digestion and the skin. If you are cold or feel sick, heat this drink and add lemon.

Elderberry Syrup: (Great for daily health, especially during the flu season, or when sick). Boil: 3 ½ cups water, 2/3 to 1 cup dried elderberries, 2 Tbs. dried or fresh ginger root, 1 tsp. cloves or clove powder. Boil 45 min. or until reduced. Cool and strain. Mix with 1 cup honey. Store in refrig. Dosage: Kids – 1 tsp; Adults – ½ to 1 Tbs. (every 2-3 hrs. if sick)

Thanks for sharing, Dana!

RECIPES/ALTERNATIVES

RECIPES

*Sugar in most recipes can be substituted with Xylitol (usually same amount) or Stevia (usually a partial amount; check Stevia package); flour can be organic; whole wheat flour's texture differs.

Fresh Pea Hummus

*This recipe contains no chickpeas. (Health.com)

1 cup frozen peas, thawed	4 Tbs. chopped walnuts
2 Tbs. fresh lemon juice	4 garlic cloves minced
½ tsp. salt	½ tsp. pepper

(My note: I would have to use less garlic for my taste.) Mix. Serve with rye crisp bread crackers. Refrigerate.

No Bake Cookies

*Etta Bruce Jordan (my aunt)

1 ½ cups Xylitol(or less)	½ cup milk
¼ lb. (stick) butter	3 Tbs. cocoa

Cook and stir these four ingredients on medium heat. When in a rolling boil, cook for 1 ½ min. Lower heat a bit; stir well. Remove from heat and add:

2 ½ cups minute oats	1 ½ tsp. vanilla

¼ cups chopped pecans (optional) or peanut butter to taste (optional)

Beat well with a big spoon, about 3-5 min. Spoon out on wax paper.

NSA Raisin Date Cookies

*Doris Brooks, MI.

Combine, then boil 3-5 min. on low heat:

1 cup raisins	½ cup chopped apples
1 cup chopped dates	1 cup water

Add: ½ cup butter; cool.
Then add:

1 egg, beaten	1 cup minute oats
½ cup chopped walnuts(or other)	1 tsp. vanilla

Mix 1 cup organic or wheat flour, 1 tsp. baking soda, and ½ tsp. salt. Mix well with wet ingredients; cover; refrigerate overnight. Drop by teaspoon on a baking sheet. Bake at 350 10-12 min.

Homemade Muesli

*Susan Rohr. Adapt all ingredients to your taste. Add other fruit. I use:

1 cup raw oats	½ chopped banana
1 apple, shredded or chopped	¼ cup milk
2 Tbs. dried raisins	2 Tbs. chopped dates
Xylitol/Stevia to taste; small, plain unsweet yogurt	chopped nuts to taste

Peach Cobbler

In a pan, slowly boil 1 can peaches (in its own juice) till peaches soften; add 1/8 cup Xylitol and water as needed to remain juicy. In pie plate or round cake pan, melt ½ stick butter. Mix together well ½ cup organic or wheat flour, ¼ tsp. baking powder, 1/8 tsp. salt, and ¼ cup Xylitol. Slowly pour flour mix over melted butter. Then pour peaches over the mix and swirl with butter knife. Bake at 375 about 30-35 min. Check and swirl 1 or 2 times.

Banana Nut Bread

1 cup Xylitol	Mix: 2 cups flour (organic,wheat)
½ cup butter(soften)	1 tsp. baking soda
1 large egg	¼ tsp. salt
3 large mashed bananas	¼ cup chopped walnuts, opt.

Cream Xylitol and butter (I use a fork). Add egg and beat well with mixer. Add bananas, then flour mix. Add nuts and beat. Pour into lined or greased bread pans. Bake 350 for 35-40 min.

Scotch Oat Cakes

*Lillias Swardson. Great with jelly, honey, etc.

3 cups oat flour	2 Tbs. Xylitol
1 cup oat bran	1 stick butter
½ tsp. salt	1 tsp.baking soda

Melt butter in 1 cup boiling water. Mix well all dry ingredients. Add wet to dry mix, stirring in well. Roll thin (like graham crackers). Cut in pieces with knife. Bake 250-275 on cookie sheet 40-45 min. (or less).

Sandwich Special

(I think some call this the Elvis sandwich because he favored this one.)

In a skillet with butter, brown both sides of 2 slices whole wheat bread (or other). Then spread 1 slice(while warm) with creamy peanut butter to taste. Put ½ sliced banana on top and drizzle with honey or agave. One of my favs, too!(Also try sliced bananas, peanut butter, and honey w/o bread.)

Peanut Butter Balls

*Lizzie Kenney, CO.

2 cups peanut butter	½ cup butter (room temp.)
1 cup honey	1 cup carob or choc. chips
2+ cups oat flour	Shredded coconut

Mix all ingredients (except coconut). (Dare you try the mixer?) Dump all out on wax paper, form into little balls, and roll in loose coconut. Put on a cookie sheet and freeze 'til hard. When ready to eat, put out a few minutes prior to soften.

Wheat Pancakes

2 cups all-purpose wheat flour	2 cups milk
4 tsp. baking powder	2 eggs

Mix in a bowl milk and eggs; mix on wax paper flour and baking powder. Stir dry into wet mix; mix well. If like thick pancakes, add ¼ cup more flour to the batter.

Alaska Blueberry Muffins

2 cups flour (organic or wheat)	1 egg
3 tsp. baking powder	1 cup milk
3 Tbs. Xylitol	3 Tbs. oil
1 tsp. salt	1 cup blueberries

Sift/mix together dry ingredients. Combine egg, milk, and oil. Add dry mix to wet; mix all at once. Stir quickly 'til just mixed. Gently fold-in blueberries. Fill muffin cups 2/3 full. Bake at 425 for 15-20 min.

Sugarless Apple Pie

Heat 1 cup frozen apple juice concentrate to boiling. Put 3 cups sliced apples in 'til they wilt. Drain, keeping juice. Thicken juice with 2 Tbs. corn starch. After juice is cooled, put apples back in the juice. Add ½ tsp. cinnamon and 2 Tbs. butter. Bake in 8-9 in. pie crusts at 400 until apples are tender and crust is golden brown. (I put foil on the edges part of that time to prevent burning.)
(Also try raw apple slices with Xylitol and cinnamon or baked apple halves with butter, Xylitol, and cinnamon.)

RECIPES-SOURCES

Internet has many natural, healthy, or low/no sugar recipe sites. Pinterest and Facebook are also sources. Try these:

MyRecipes.com

FoodBabe.com

Nutritionella.com

HealthyMama.com

Health.com/health/recipes

Recipes According to Elle

My Fitness Pal

WellnessMomma.com

ALTERNATIVES

1. Dr. Joseph Mercola (alternative medicine proponent): How to Keep Your Home Clean Naturally
2. Spafromscratch.com/homemade-deodorant
3. Budget101.com/household items
4. How Toxic Are Your Household Cleaning Supplies? (Organic Consumer's Association) This has a great list of safer cleaners, some homemade.
5. Guide to Less Toxic Products (Two year Canadian study, revised 2011 from 2004) Excellent and very comprehensive guide to alternatives.
6. EWG (Environmental Working Group) offers many alternatives to chemicals.

7. "Eight Household Cleaning Agents to Avoid," offers healthier, non-toxic alternatives for furniture polish, rug deodorizer, mothball replacement, whitening scouring powder, glass cleaner, etc. (i.e. Rug deodorizer-Sprinkle dry carpet with baking soda. Wait 15 minutes and vacuum. May repeat if need.)

8. Homemade Deodorant (Mercola.com): 3 Tbs. virgin coconut oil; 2 Tbs. shea butter; 3 Tbs. baking soda, 2 Tbs. cornstarch; 5 drops essential oil (peppermint, spearmint, lavender, orange, lemon,vanilla). Place a half-pint glass jar in the middle of a small pot of water (like a double boiler effect). Bring the water to a simmer. Add coconut oil and shea butter to jar and let melt. Turn off the heat and add soda and starch. Stir till smooth. Add essential oil. This will liquefy in warmer temps and solidify in cooler.

9. "Clorox VS Peroxide." Becky Ramsey, physician's wife from Indiana. She is an advocate of peroxide. Cleaner: 50/50 mix of water and peroxide. Spray countertops to kill germs; use in bathroom to disinfect. Laundry: Add 1 cup peroxide instead of bleach to whiten clothes. (Blood stains-pour directly on soiled spot. Soak 1+ minute. Rub and rinse with cold water.) Bathroom: Urine on floor under the toilet? Spray or wipe with peroxide. Smell is gone and bacteria eliminated. Check her site for peroxide use with toothache, sinus infection, infections and cuts, foot fungus, canker sores, white teeth, and

more.(There is controversy about the effectiveness of peroxide, so do your own research.)

10. For general cleaning: white vinegar and water. Also use hydrogen peroxide, lemon juice, borax, and baking soda. Seventh Generation and other healthier alternatives may be purchased at health food stores. Walmart and Target are beginning to carry organic and fragrance-free products, as are other stores in communities. If you have a healthier product, and see the words *parfum*, *perfume*, or *fragrance* in its list of ingredients, the whole product has been contaminated with myriad toxins.

MY PRODUCTS

Over the years, many people have asked what I use. I am not endorsing any company or store, just fragrance-free, organic, or homemade products. I have a chemical-free home, but I do use some pure essential oils in my products and in my diffuser.

I would not think of using a plug-in or wall- mounted deodorizer in my home! And I cannot believe stores are still stocking them. I buy the 2 oz. fingertip spray bottles ($.99 at Walmart in travel sample section). Fill it almost full of water (preferably filtered). Then add 10-15 drops of pure essential oil. Try peppermint, spearmint, vanilla, orange, lemon, lavender, and others from health food stores. Shake, spray, and enjoy—without the toxins of other deodorizers.

For glass and window cleaning, kitchen and bath counter tops, get a spray bottle. Fill half to three-quarters with water, then finish filling with white vinegar. Shake well, spray, and wipe with a dry cloth or paper towel.

Laundry products are so important because clothes cover the entire body. Since skin is our biggest organ, everything put on the skin absorbs readily into the bloodstream and is constantly inhaled by the mouth and nose. I use the #1 recommended by allergists, dermatologists, and pediatricians: ALL FREE. During the sickest part of MCS, Seventh Generation and All Free were all I could tolerate. I never, ever use fabric softener (see PART II: FYI section). Vinegar is all I use in the rinse cycle (can put in softener dispenser, too). My daughters use pure essential oils for some non-toxic fragrance. One puts it in her rinse cycle; one adds it (5+ drops) to her All Free wash.

Soaps, somewhat like laundry products, affect the skin. Kiss My Face makes a pure olive oil soap for sensitive skin. Now I enjoy Zum, Dessert Essence, and other high quality soaps with pure essential oils. Lemon scents are among my favorites.

I put nothing on my body that I cannot eat! Coconut oil (refined for no smell, unrefined for coconut smell) is my best friend. Wet the skin first, then rub small amounts all over the body parts that can be reached. Some people keep their jar in the shower to apply while still wet. (I use 1-2 Tbs. a day. This and aloe vera gel are great for minor female irritations.) Almond oil is also one I like. And I've heard olive oil with some essential oil (to avoid smelling like olive oil) is a good lotion. Avocado and jojoba oils moisturize well.

For headaches, I try rubbing the temples with peppermint or lavender oil in a coconut oil base. I also use acupressure, a method my mom taught me and that I've used with my girls for years. With fingertips, apply pressure at the base of the skull, left and right of the spine top. Press for about a minute. Then apply pressure outside each eye, bit below where the eyebrow ends. The nose is next. Press at the lower base of the nose, on its left and right sides, where the nose joins the face. Last are the hands; do one at a time. In the webbed area between the thumb and index finger, apply pressure on top and underneath using thumb and index finger of opposite hand. Find the tender area(s) and press for about a minute.

For virus, flu, or sinus infections, I like to use Thieves, Purification, or Eucalyptus in my essential oil diffuser. I treat with the following supplements: Vitamin C, Vitamin D3, oreganol oil (under the tongue then rinse with water as it's a hot oil), and elderberry syrup (I like Sambucus brand.) I also use colloidal silver and Natural Factors lung, respiratory, and sinus blend tablet. Remember: I am not trying to play doctor here; I'm merely sharing what I use since I cannot and do not like to use chemicals.

For deodorant, I use white vinegar and essential oil/water mix. First, I wet a jumbo cotton ball with vinegar, then some water and rub one arm pit. Then add a bit more vinegar and water and rub the other arm pit.

Vinegar is a natural disinfectant so kills the odor-causing bacteria. (It takes a few days to notice a difference.) Let dry. Then I spray my homemade fragrance (2 oz. fingertip spray bottle filled with water and 8-10 drops of my favorite essential oil). This is similar to my homemade room deodorizers but not as strong for it can sting the underarm's sensitive skin. I sometimes use a deodorant made from Dead Sea salt.

For teeth, I floss almost nightly, use an organic fluoride-free toothpaste, then follow that with homemade salt/soda mix. Since I've been using the salt/soda, I've had better dental check-ups.

I'm going to try Dana's soda and vinegar hair-cleaning system soon, but I've been using fragrance-free shampoos and conditioners from health food stores, which is where one daughter gets hair gels; I use a bit of coconut oil to scrunch my curls. These stores also have hair dyes and many other personal products. (I've been using Dana's white vinegar hair rinse and like it.)

For general cleaning, I usually use vinegar and water. I also like Dr. Bronner's Sal Suds and Seventh Generation products. I use these two items to clean my floors, counter tops...almost everything in my house. I see if Walmart or Target has products I use; if not, I go to health food stores. For floors I use a gallon or so of water and 1/8 to ¼ cup white vinegar. I damp mop my wood and laminate wood floors by squeezing out excess water or by mopping them after I've used up the wet on the tile floors.

To clean the oven and bathtubs, I first wet with water what I'm cleaning, then sprinkle or add baking soda to make a paste or cover. Let soak 1 hr. (tub)-3 hrs. (oven), scrub, and rinse with wash cloth. Bad grime requires another application. (EWG cites very similar-sprinkle a liberal amount of baking soda, spray with water, wait 8 hrs. for an oven and scrape).

I stress again: READ THE INGREDIENTS. Watch fragrances and other chemicals. You have one body for this lifetime, as does your child. When it wears out or is ravaged by chemicals, you are in trouble, as I found out over 20 years ago. All I know is I was a very sick, toxic person who was told I had 5-7 years. That was in 1995. Praise God and the healthier route He gave me to follow.

NOTEWORTHY ADDITIONAL INFORMATION

1. Three principle routes of exposure (pathway by which a chemical enters the body): SKIN, LUNGS, MOUTH.

   <u>Skin</u> (absorption)-What we put on the skin often passes through the skin to the blood, then is carried to various organs including the brain, liver, and kidneys where it may have immediate or long term effects. The scalp is especially absorbent.

   <u>Lungs</u>(inhalation)-Lung tissue is very thin. It allows passage of not only oxygen but also other chemicals directly into the blood stream. Once in the blood, it passes to the heart and then is distributed to other organs without passing to the liver to detox. Aerosol sprays and airborne ingredients in personal-care products and house-cleaning products become part of the air we breathe at home, work, or school.

   <u>Mouth</u> (ingestion to digestive tract)-Chemicals on or in food we eat and drink can be ingested. Children, who put their hands everywhere (including the mouth) or chew on various objects, are likely to ingest chemicals. Ingested chemicals absorb anywhere along the digestive tract, but the major site is the small intestine. The type exposure can affect the impact a chemical has. The greater the absorption, the greater the potential for a chemical to exert a toxic effect.

2. EPA 1991 Study-A room containing an air freshener had high levels of a carcinogen (p-dichlorobenzene) and ethanol (on EPA hazardous waste list and a cause of CNS disorders). (My note: And they are still in stores selling like hotcakes??!!) [xli]

3. Lysol isn't required to list ingredients.(And were difficult to find!) Some of its ingredients include: etharo (flammable); alkyldimethyl benzylammonia chloride (irritates respiratory function and asthma, and is a hazardous gas when mixed with products that contain bleach); denatured alcohol (respiratory irritant, CNS depression, eye and mucous membrane irritant); isopropyl alcohol. Caution: Avoid using in enclosed areas for long periods of time. In 1911, poisoning by drinking Lysol was the most common means of suicide in Australia.[xlii] Lysol is a chemical disinfectant that the EPA classifies as a pesticide. Of the 148 ingredients for Lysol's 96 products, EWG's rating was A=0; B=11; C=9; D=28; and F=48. [xliii]Research dangers of your cleaning products.

4. Vinegar-Age old disinfectant; Purdue University recently approved it as a deodorizer/disinfectant. I read that but can't find it online now. What happened? Many facilities do use it as a disinfectant.

5. Bleach-MO Health Dept. told me if you can smell it, your solution is too strong. Use 1 part bleach to 100 parts water.

6. According to the FDA, fragrances cause 30% of all allergic reactions and all asthmatics can develop respiratory symptoms when exposed to perfume. The average North American uses 17-21 scented products a day! Of 2,983 chemicals tested by the FDA, 844 toxic substances were found. They can cause cancer, birth defects, CNS disorders and are linked to asthma, allergies, and liver/kidney/neurological damage.[xliv]

7. November 11, 2010 newsletter from St. Jude Children's Research Hospital: More than 5,700 children are now being treated by St. Jude. Thousands more will develop cancer this year (2010).

8. Online, Google "Dangers of Fragrances."

9. Avoid carrageenan (extract from seaweed used as a thickening agent, usually in dairy and meat products). It causes gastrointestinal issues, inflammation, and cancer.

10. Terrazzo floors: eco-friendly floors (greenwiseflooring.com)

11. Fragrance ingredients are considered "Trade Secrets" under the U.S. Fair Packaging and Labeling Act.

12. Beware of the words *natural, green, botanical, and eco-friendly.* Often, manufacturers of hazardous products dress-up their containers with words and pretty flower pictures; they play on our desire for more natural products.

13. *Unscented* vs *fragrance-free: Unscented* is misleading and means no fragrance has been added to

the product; however, some of its ingredients may be scented (to cover the unpleasant smells of other ingredients, as a rep of Secret unscented deodorant informed me on the phone.) *Fragrance-free* is supposed to be a guarantee of no fragrance/scent in the product.

14. Oxyclean is made of mainly baking soda and washing soda. Get the Free type to ensure no fragrance. The one with blue crystals has a scent or smell.

15. EWG (one of largest environmental groups in the U.S.) studied and rated (for environmental health and safety)many household cleaning products. A,B,C,D, and F were the ratings, with A being safest and F being least safe. Among the A's were: Dr. Bronner's Sal Suds, Ecover products, Arm & Hammer Baking and Washing Soda, Darth Friendly products, Heinz white distilled vinegar, Whole Foods brands, Green Shield Organics, and Aspen Clean. Some F's included: 409; Walmart Great Value glass and general purpose; Ajax; Clorox: Green Works; Pledge; Simple Green; Soft Scrub; Mr. Clean; LA's; Fabuloso; Endust; Swiffer; CVC cleaners; Windex; and most Lysol products rated in this category(except for Lysol Brand III disinfectant and all purpose cleaner 4-in-1 spray, orange and Brand III 4-in-1 all purpose cleaner; its lemon breeze received a B rating).[xlv]

SUMMARIES

Following are brief summaries of helpful, informative articles. Please Google them on the internet and read the articles in their entirety. I went overload on fragrances because they are most deceptive. Most of us do not know they are toxic and dangerous. We can read food labels (fragrances have none), and we know pesticides, exhaust, and cigarette smoke are toxic.

CANCER

American Cancer Society, 2014.
In the U.S., 15,780 (birth-19 yrs.) each year are diagnosed with cancer. (36 a day in 2010; 43 a day in 2014!) ACS estimates 10,450 new cases (Age 0-14) with 1,350 deaths and 5,330 new cases (ages 15-19) with 610 deaths in 2014. Before age 20, 1 in 285 children are expected to have cancer. They report that cancer is the second leading cause of death (ages 5-14).

"The 'C' Word – Better Nutrition." Dr. Emily A. Kane, ND, Lac. April 2015. www.betternutrition.com.
Most experts think cancer starts with a single damaged cell that receives several hits (man-made chemicals, natural poisons, physical trauma, and emotional stress). Genetics plays a small role; environmental pollution is the #1 risk factor. Top 10 cancer-fighting foods: beans; carotenoid-rich fruits and veggies (deep green, orange, yellow); cruciferous veggies (broccoli, cabbage, kale, cauliflower); fiber-rich foods (beans, fruits, veggies, whole grains); fish (coldwater like salmon, trout, snapper); garlic; green tea; mushrooms (maitake, reishi, shiitake); nuts and seeds; yogurt (organic,

plain from grass-fed animals). Helpful supplements: green tea, melatonin, Vitamin D3, medicinal mushrooms.

"Cancer in Children and Adolescents." American Cancer Society, 2014. www.cancer.org/acs/.
Predominant cancers of ages 0-19 yrs. are leukemia (26%), cancers of the brain and CNS (18%), and lymphoma (14%). As of January 2010, there are (approximately) 379,112 cancer survivors, ages 0-19 yrs. "It is known that the process of development occurring in immature cells and organisms renders them more vulnerable to toxic exposures than mature cells, and it is therefore important to minimize exposure to environmental agents with potential cancer-causing effects."

"Causes and Prevention: National Cancer Institute." www.cancer.gov/cancertopics/prevention.
Prevention: antioxidants, calcium, cancer vaccines, cruciferous veggies, garlic, tea, Vitamin D, physical activity, surgery, statins, pap & HPV testing, HPV vaccines. (My note: No mention of chemicals, except use of antioxidants. And statins?)

"Cancer Prevention: 7 Tips to Reduce Your Risk." Mayo Clinic. Dec. 12, 2012. www.mayoclinic.org.
Mayo did acknowledge that there are conflicting reports about cancer prevention. Four of their seven include (1) Don't use tobacco and avoid all second -hand smoke. (2) Eat a healthy diet with plenty of veggies and fruit, little fat and alcohol. (3) Maintain a healthy weight and be physically active, with a minimum of 150 minutes a week moderate aerobic activity. (4) Protect yourself from the sun.

(My note: Again, not one mention about avoiding chemicals, which contain many carcinogens.)

"Does Sugar Promote Heart Disease and Cancer?" Dr. Joseph Mercola. March and December 2013. Mercola.com.
More than 1,660,290 new cancer cases are projected in 2013. An estimated 580,350 will die from the disease according to the American Cancer Society. He believes the root cause to be a diet high in sugars and processed foods. Sugar decreases the function of your immune system, and tumor cells thrive on sugar (sweets, breads, pasta, grains...)

The Gerson Therapy. Dr. Max Gerson. Pp. 18-20.
In 1958, Dr. Max Gerson was the first physician ever to state that cancer was caused by multiple interdependent factors. A minimum of 49 stressors exist. Most critical are the number and types of carcinogenic hits, their frequency, and their intensity. Taken from medical, environmental, and scientific literature and experiences, some of the 49 stressors include: sunlight's ultraviolet rays; atmospheric cosmic rays and x-rays; sick building syndrome; microwave oven radiation; pesticide/herbicide residues; industrial toxins; drinking/bathing in polluted, chlorinated, and fluoridated water; tobacco and smoking; hormonal therapies; immune-suppressive drugs; consuming irradiated foods; ingesting food additives; dental metals, fillings, root canals; use of street, prescription, and nonprescription drugs; diet or nutritional deficiencies; synthetic nonfood consumption; chronic mental/physical stress; destructive negative emotions; intestinal toxicity; parasites; blocked detox; free radicals; and genetic predisposition. (My note:

Check out the remaining 26+. Now, almost 60 years later, we have a chemical society. Fragrance alone overlaps several of the 49 stressors.)

The Gerson Therapy, Revised. The Proven Nutritional Program for Cancer and Other Illnesses. Charlotte Gerson and Morton Walker, D.P.M. Kensington Publishing Corp., 2001, 2006.

Dr. Max Gerson was a top authority in the study of natural treatment of cancer. In the 1940's, 1 in 16 people had cancer; in 2006, it was 1 in 3, nearing 1 in 2. He felt two causes of cancer were deficiency and toxicity. He identified three steps in cancer development: (1) 1st Step (initiation): The hits produce free radicals which set up a pathological process that damages the cells' DNA. The liver plays a vital role in cancer formation, simultaneously initiating carcinogenesis and neutralizing it. (2) 2nd Step (promotion): The liver's neutralization may not be up to par and a damaged cell alters its pattern of mitosis (normal cell division). It begins to divide voluminously. (3) 3rd Step (progression): The tumor attempts to build itself a blood supply for sustained nourishment. Tumorous invasion of surrounding tissues may take place.

Medicine and Science in Sports and Exercise. 2003.
…more than 100 epidemiologic studies on the role of physical activity and cancer prevention…30-60 minutes a day of moderate to vigorous physical activity is needed. The adrenaline helps circulate natural killer immune cells into tumors in the lung, liver, and skin or to help lower the risk of cancer later in life.

National Children's Cancer Society. Topeka, KS and St. Louis, MO. Sept. 2010. www.chilcren-cancer.org. 1-800-532-6459.
Primary mission: to provide direct financial and in-kind assistance to children with cancer and their families. There are 170,000 + survivors of childhood cancer in the U.S. Cancer is the leading cause of death by disease among U.S. children ages 1 to 14. Most common childhood cancers: leukemia, lymphoma, and brain cancer.

"No Escape: Tests Find Toxic Fire Retardants in Mothers. EWG. Aug. 4, 1914. www.ewg.org/.
A study by EWG scientists and Duke University scientists found a biomarker of cancer-causing fire retardant in babies of all 22 mothers and 26 children tested. Children had five times the level of this biomarker than their moms.

President's Cancer Panel: Environmentally Caused Cancers. (Also: "Grievous Harm-The Report of the President's Cancer Panel.")Environmental Health News, May 7, 2010 – a 240 page report.
The President's Cancer Panel reported, "The true burden of environmentally induced cancers has been grossly underestimated," and strongly urged action to reduce people's widespread exposure to carcinogens. The panel advised President Obama,"…to use the power of your office to remove the carcinogens and other toxins from our food, water, and air that needlessly increase health care costs, cripple our nation's productivity, and devastate American lives." Only a few hundred of the 80,000 + chemicals in use in the U.S. have been tested for safety. (My note: This report was in 2010. The panel was

composed of three members, two of whom are distinguished scientists or physicians. I didn't even know we have a President's Cancer Panel. Has there been improvement, or was the panel's research and advice ignored?)

"Rise in Childhood Cancers Parallels Toxic Chemical Proliferation." Environmental News Service, Jan. 26, 2011. www.ens-newswire.com.
Bi-partisan legislation introduced in Congress to help communities determine if there's a connection between clusters of cancer, birth defects and other diseases, and contaminants in the surrounding environment.

FRAGRANCE

I have targeted fragrance because it is so deceptive. It smells good but is toxic— thus its name, Sweet Poison (in the environmental circle). Pure essential oils are a much healthier choice, although they bother some people who have allergies, asthma, or chemical sensitivities.

CDC's Fragrance-Free Policy. Spring 2010.
CDC (Center for Disease Control and Prevention) is committed to providing all CDC workers a safe place of employment and will take action to keep the workplace free of recognized hazards. Therefore, in 2010, CDC issued the "Indoor Environmental Quality Policy." It applied to all CDC workers at all facilities; it banned the use of fragrance in the workplace. CDC was praised for its landmark decision to acknowledge the harmful effects of fragrance and other chemicals. (Complete story and policy: CDC Indoor Environmental Quality policy). The story began in 2001 with a plug-in air freshener. Non-permissible products include all scented or fragranced products: incense, candles, fragrance-emitting devises, plug-in or spray air deodorizers, toilet blocks, personal care products including colognes and perfumes, and hair products—even essential oils. Employees are to arrive at work as fragrance-free as possible; avoid using scented detergents and fabric softeners. (My note: To me, this spoke volumes! Our authority on disease prevention and control eliminated fragrance. Think about it, Folks.)

"Could Scented Candles Kill You?" Daily Mail. Sept. 2, 2015.

Research has shown some scented candles produce smoke laced with almost as many toxins as cigarettes.

"Eleven Taken to Hospital after Perfume Sickens Students." New Hampshire *Union Leader,* Sept. 12, 2008. (Also: "Fragrance Sickens Several Men and 11 Students.")
A perfume bottle spilled on the school bus ride home. The scent made men pass out. Eleven were checked out at the hospital.

Fragrance: A Growing Health and Environmental Hazard. 1991 EPA study by Klaw Ferlow, May 2008.
www.positirehealth.com.
The skin, our body's largest organ, absorbs fragrance chemicals by direct application, by contact with fragrance items (laundry, clothes), and by exposure to air containing fragrance. Ninety-five per cent of the fragrance chemicals are petroleum derivatives with many of the same chemicals as cigarette smoke— but there are no regulations for the fragrance industry. (My note: For over 25 years, we have been that industry's victims). In 2008, the estimated annual sale of scented products was 47.15 billion (My note: Big time! Think they want to lose that revenue?) Health condition estimates from fragrance pollutants: allergies— 40-50 million; skin allergies— 1.7 to 4.1% of population; rhinitis (nasal)—40 million; chronic sinus—35 million; asthma—over 20.3 million; chemical sensitivities—6 to 16% of population; chronic lung disease—15 million; migraine headaches—28 million.

Fragrance and Health. Louise A. Kosta. H.E.A.L., Atlanta, GA, 1998.
One in five (now one in three) Americans may experience harm from fragrance exposure. This book shows WHO is susceptible to these adverse affects, WHY they are, WHERE the harmful fragrance exposures are, and WHAT harmful properties fragrance materials may have.

Fragrance: Emerging Health and Environmental Concerns. Betty Bridges. Fragranced Products Information Network, Amelia, VA, April and Sept. 2002. Flavours and Fragrance, John Wiley & Sons, Ltd. www.onlinelibrary.wiley.com. Great list of references. Also contains regulations from different countries, health concerns (skin, respiratory, neurological, and systemic effects), and environmental concerns.

"Fresh Scent Hides Toxic Secrets." Washington Toxics, Lisa Stiffler, adapted from *Seattle Post-Intelligencer.* July 24, 2008. www.watoxics.org.
The scented fabric sheet makes shirts and socks smell flowery fresh and clean. That plug-in air freshener fills homes with inviting fragrances of apple, cinnamon, or a country garden. But these common household items are potentially exposing family and friends to dangerous chemicals, a University of Washington study has found.

"Heavenly Scents or Toxic Fumes—Are Your Fragrances Healing or Killing You?" John P. Thomas. *Health Impact News.* Posted by site admin., May 28, 2014.

Healthimpactnews.com. (*Alternative Health.* "Fragrance: A Growing Health and Environmental Hazard; see also "Conscious Choice: Smells Can Make You Sick." Lynn Lawson.)

Naturally fragrant pure essential oils can heal, but manufactured scents can make people sick and even cause death. Petroleum and coal tar comprise about 95% of large corporations' fragrances. Toxic solvents are added so they have a high VOC content to make airborne fragrance molecules adhere to clothes, skin, hair, etc. for hours, days, or months. (My note: One closet in my house of two years STILL smells from the previous owner's fragrances.) Daily exposure to these chemical fragrances creates a chemical dependency (addiction). As with other addictions, more and stronger are needed—and fragrance addicts feel they're not fully dressed for the day without their fragrance. Many chemicals in synthetic fragrances are known to be carcinogenic (cancerous) and neurotoxic. However, the fragrance industry is not required to prove safety. "Artificial fragrances are more like gasoline than flowers," said one of their reports. Another said he and his insurance company had spent thousands over a few years to treat a sinus allergy that was caused by their choice of laundry products.

"Making Sense of Scents." Compiled by the late Julia Kendall, borrowing from Irene Wilkenfeld's "Fragrance Facts." www.scents4youteam.com.

As early as 1986, the National Academy of Sciences targeted six categories of chemicals for neurotoxicity testing priority: fragrances, insecticides, heavy metals, solvents, food additives, and certain air pollutants. They said 95% of chemicals used in fragrances are synthetic petroleum compounds, some of which were neurotoxic, hazard waste chemicals, and causes of cancer and birth defects. National Institute of Occupational Safety and Health reports that 884 toxic substances were identified in a partial list of 2,983 chemicals used in the fragrance industry; many are capable of causing cancer, birth defects, CNS disorders, breathing and allergic reactions, and multiple chemical sensitivities. Toulene was detected in every fragrance sample by EPA in a 1991 report. It triggers asthma attacks, causes asthma, and is carcinogenic.

"Perfume: Cupid's Arrow or Poison Dart." Joint release by Cancer Prevention Coalition and Environmental Health Network, Dr. Samuel S. Epstein and Amy Marsh. Feb. 7, 2000. www.prnewswire.com.
Is your Valentine gift of perfume a bottle of toxic chemicals? Currently the fragrance industry is virtually unregulated. An analysis of Calvin Klein's *Eternity* revealed 41 ingredients, some known to be toxic to the skin, respiratory tract, nervous and reproductive systems and others known to be carcinogens.

"Scented Products Emit a Bouquet of VOC's." Carol Poters, *Environment Health Perspectives*. Jan. 1, 2011.
The FDA requires the term *fragrance* on personal care items but does NOT require the ingredients of fragrances. A single fragrance can contain a mix of hundreds of chemicals. (FDA Code of Federal Regulations, Title 21, Part 701. Cosmetic Labeling. Dec. 2010.) Claudia Miller, allergist and immunologist at University of Texas Health

Science Center, "…strongly suggest that we need to find unscented alternatives…"

"Secret Chemicals in Perfumes—Are about to Be Unbottled ." Amy Westervelt, *The Guardian,* Oct. 15, 2014. www.theguardian.com.
Women's Voices for the Earth has pressured S.C. Johnson Co., and finally it is exposing (via its website) ingredients (especially fragrance) in its products. Clorox plans to do the same. Expert Anne M. Steinemann found in a 2009 study that 30.5 % of the U.S. population reported skin irritation and/or headaches when exposed to scented products.

"Secret Chemicals Revealed in Celebrity Perfumes, Teen Body Sprays." EWG, May 12, 2010. www.ewg.org.
Studies of hidden toxic chemicals in perfumes come on the heels of a recent President's Cancer Panel report, which sounded the alarm over the understudied and largely unregulated toxic chemicals used daily by millions of Americans. Fragrances mentioned with secret chemicals that could trigger allergic reactions, disrupt hormones, and cause asthma, headaches, and contact dermatitis included: Calvin Klein's *Eternity*; Abercrombie & Fitch's *Fierce*; Hannah Montana's *Secret Celebrity*; Brittany Spears' *Curious*; American Eagle's *Seventy-Seven*; Giorgio Armeni's *Acqua DiGlo* , Halle Berry's *Halle,* House of Quicksilver's *Quicksilver*, and Jennifer Lopez's *J Lo Glow*, along with others.

"Students Go to Hospital after Someone Sprays AXE Body Spray in School." *Business Insider.* Saranya Kapur. Nov. 1, 2013. www.businessinsider.com.

AXE was sprayed in a sixth grade class, and eight Brooklyn kids had to be taken to the hospital.

** "Sweet Poison: The Dangers of Perfume." Julia Kendall, ref. Lance Wallace, EPA, excerpts from MSDS Health Hazard Information. Oct. 16, 2003 and same info in 2015. www.ecomall.com/greenshopping.

The 20 most common chemicals found in 31 fragrance products (including dish and dishwasher detergents, detergents and fabric softeners, cologne and perfume, deodorant, soap, lotion, hairspray, shampoo, air deodorizers, nail enamel) in an EPA test in 1991 reveal the following (first five most commonly used):

(1) Benzyl acetate: carcinogenic; irritates eyes and respiratory; systemic effects if absorbed through skin. Do not flush to sewer.

(2) Benzyl alcohol: irritating to upper respiratory; CNS depressant; headache; nausea; dizziness; death from respiratory failure.

(3) Limonene: carcinogenic; eye and skin irritant; damaging to immune system. Do not inhale. (My note: We inhale fragrances!)

(4) Linalool: narcotic; respiratory; attracts bees (My note: I've read pesticides are added to fragrance. I can often smell pesticide in fragrances, especially deodorizers.); CNS disorder.

(5) A-terpineol: CNS and respiratory depression; headache; very irritating to mucous membranes; pneumonitis (lung aspiration – even fatal edema). Prevent repeated or prolonged skin contact.

(6) Acetone: on EPA and other Hazardous Waste lists; CNS depressant; incoordination; drowsiness; coma in severe exposure.

(7) Benzaldehyde: narcotic; CNS depressant; damaging to immune system; irritant to throat, eyes, skin, lungs and GI tract; may cause kidney damage.

(8) Ethanol: on EPA Hazardous Waste list; fatigue; eye and upper respiratory irritant; drowsiness; impaired vision; CNS disorders.

(9) Ethyl acetate: on EPA Hazardous Waste list; narcotic; irritates eyes and respiratory; headaches; stupor; damage to liver and kidneys; dry and cracking skin.

(10)   Camphor: CNS stimulant; irritates eyes, nose, throat; dizziness; confusion; twitching muscles; confusion. Avoid inhaling.

(11)   Methylene chloride: carcinogen; banned by FDA in 1988 (no enforcement due to Trade Secret laws that protect chemical fragrance industry); EPA and other Hazardous Waste lists; stored in body fat; CNS disorder; headache; giddiness; stupor; irritability; fatigue; tingling in limbs.

(12)   A-pinene: sensitizer(damaging to immune system)

(13)   G-terpinene: asthma; CNS disorders

(Unable to obtain MSDS for: 8-cineole; b-citronellol; b-myrcene; nerol; ocimene; b-phenethyl alcohol; a-terpinolene.)

"Sweet Poison: What Your Nose Can't Tell You about the Dangers of Perfume." Enviroknow's Health and Environment Resource Center. Intro by Andrea DesJardins, 1997. Members.aol.com/chemxpose. mem Chemical fragrance is everywhere. One fragrant product may contain up to 600 of the 5,000 chemicals used. Studies show it to cause health effects, mainly of the skin, lungs, and brain. Children are even more susceptible than adults to the effects of these chemicals, yet fragrances are added to nearly every baby product on the market! Parents wearing and using these chemical scented products may well be poisoning the air their children breathe. Exposure can result in difficulty concentrating, learning disabilities, hyperactive behavior, and even growth retardation. There also may be headaches (especially migraines), sneezing, watery eyes, sinus problems, nausea, and difficulty swallowing. (My note: Other studies also point to cancer since several ingredients are carcinogens. Notated in this section.)

"Workers Hospitalized from Perfume." The Associated Press, July 30, 2009. www.highbeam.com
About 150 people were sickened. Fire officials suspected carbon monoxide or other toxin, but perfume was to

blame. Bank of America call center in Ft. Worth, TX co-worker sprayed perfume. Perfume not identified at press time.

DEODORIZERS

"Air Freshener Chemicals and Their Health Effects." Air Purifier Basics, 2004. airpurifierbasics.com.
People buy chemical air fresheners to improve the air quality in their homes. They actually make it unhealthy or unsafe. If you have eye irritation, headaches, or other strange symptoms—and are using air fresheners, stop using them for some time and observe how you or your family feel. Air fresheners contain limonene (a skin, mouth, and eye irritant which can cause dizziness and incoordination). It's carcinogenic (cancer causing) and is damaging to the immune system. Its petroleum distillates can irritate or damage the lungs. Toulene is also a carcinogenic and causes fatigue and confusion. Carcinogenic benzene compounds and the hormone disruptor phthalate are in many fresheners. They contain many other chemicals as well.

"Air Fresheners—Silent Menace." Andrea DesJardins, 2008-2010. silentmenace.com/home.
In no way does a chemically-scented fragrance or aerosol (propelled by butane, propane, or other toxin) create an indoor environment of fresh air. Reports of chemical air-freshener dangers are making the news. An MSN article stated that being exposed to air "freshener" chemicals one time a week can increase asthma

symptom development by 71% and increase the risk of pulmonary illness. There are warnings about inhaling the vapors. Acetone and propane are cardiovascular or blood toxicants; liver, kidney, and gastrointestinal toxicants; neurotoxicant; skin and respiratory toxicants. Acetone is also on EPA's Hazardous Waste list. Butane is a neurotoxicant. Glade (and other) plug-ins and car oils contain perfumes (with many unlabeled toxic ingredients) and amorphous fumed silica which can cause a non reversible and fatal lung disease. The MSDS warns it can be an irritation to nose, throat, and respiratory tract. Airwick is vaguer.

Georgia Police: "Woman Dies after Exposure to an Odor at McDonald's." CNN, Sept. 8, 2011. www.cnn.com/2011.
One woman died and at least eight other people were hospitalized after being exposed to an odor at a McDonald's restaurant....happened in a restroom.

"Ingredients in Deodorizers." Clinical Toxicology of Commercial Products. Gosselin, Smith, and Hodge, 1984. EPA, TSCA, Sect. 21, 2015.
1984: ethyl/isopropyl alcohol, glycol ethers, perfume, water, propellants, petroleum distillates, metazene, ethanol, cellasolve acetate, aluminum chlorhydrol (see article for compete list).   2015: absorbents, oxidizers, surfactants, fragrances, aerosol propellants, solvents, benzene, formaldehyde, toluene, terpenes, styrene, phthalate esters (see article for complete list). Some ingredients are KNOWN carcinogens. Some are known to have a wide range of immediate and long-term toxic

effects on vital organs. (My note: Supermarkets have huge displays of these toxic sprays!)

LAUNDRY

"Chemical Emissions from Residential Dryer Vents During Use of Fragranced Laundry Products." Dr. Anne C. Steinemann, Lisa G. Gallagher, Amy L. Davis, and Ian C. MacGregor. Springer Science and Business Media. *Air Quality, Atmosphere, and Health.* March 1, 2013. www.national-toxic-encephalopathy-foundation.org.

Air vented from machines using top-selling scented laundry detergent and dryer sheets contains hazardous chemicals. More than 25 VOC's were found, including seven hazardous air pollutants, two of which (acetaldehyde and benzene) are classified as CARCINOGENS by the EPA. Dr. Steinemann noted that emissions "…coming out of a smokestack or tailpipe…" are regulated but dryer vents are not. She recommended using laundry products without fragrance or scent.

"Chemicals Found in Fabric Softeners." U.S. EPA, Lance Wallace. Oct. 7, 1998. Compiled by Julia Kendall from MSDS (material safety data sheets).

Fabric softeners, like other fragrant products, contain petrochemicals which can adversely affect the CNS (brain and spine). CNS exposures include disorientation, dizziness, headaches, numbness, pain in the neck or spine, blurred vision. CNS disorders: Alzheimer's, ADD, Dementia, MCS, MS, Parkinson's, seizures, strokes, SIDS. (See article for much more info.) Chemicals found and their effects:

(1) Alpha terpineol: CNS disorders; headaches; mucosal irritant

(2) Benzyl acetate: carcinogenic; eye and respiratory irritant

(3) Benzyl alcohol: CNS disorders; respiratory irritant and possible failure; headache; nausea

(4) Camphor: CNS disorders; EPA Hazardous Waste list; eye, nose, throat irritant. Avoid inhaling.

(5) Chloroform: carcinogenic; EPA Hazardous Waste list; kidney/liver damage with over exposure. Avoid contact with skin, eyes, and clothing.

(6) Ethanol: on EPA Hazardous Waste list; CNS disorders; fatigue; eye and upper respiratory irritant

(7) Ethyl acetate: narcotic; EPA Hazardous Waste list; eye and respiratory irritant; may cause anemia and damage to liver and kidneys

(8) Limonene: carcinogenic; skin and eye irritant. Do not inhale.

(9) Linalool: narcotic; CNS disorders; respiratory disturbances

(10)   Pentane: dermatitis; respiratory tract irritant; headache; dizziness; vomiting; harmful if inhaled; extremely flammable. Keep from heat and avoid vapors.

"Fabric Softeners and Your Liver." Nicole Cutler, LAC. Aug. 12, 2011. Liversupport.com/fabric-softeners. According to the Allergy and Environmental Health Association, both liquid and dryer sheet fabric softeners are the most toxic products produced for daily household use. Of the nine (9) chemicals the liver has to filter, three are carcinogens, six are nervous system toxins, and two damage the liver. (My note: Vinegar, Anyone?)

"Fabric Softener Toxicity Investigated." Profile by Treesha de France. "Toxicity of Fabric Softener Emissions," Rosalind C. and Julius H. Anderson, Anderson Laboratories, Inc. W. Hartford, VT, *Journal of Toxicology and Environmental Health.*
Tests demonstrated there is a toxicological explanation for the eye irritations and breathing difficulties (and other irritations) that have been reported by some individuals after exposure to fabric softener emissions.

"The Toxic Danger of Fabric Softener and Dryer Sheets." Compiled by Julia Kendall from industry-generated MSDS and from EPA's "Identification of Polar VOC's in Consumer Products," Lance Wallace. Jan. 13, 2012, Sixwise.com. and Oct. 2013, https://essentialsolutions.wordpress.com.
Although they make your clothes feel soft and smell fresh, fabric softener and dryer sheets are some of the most toxic products around. The chemicals are pungent and strong smelling, so strong they require use of heavy extra fragrances to cover up smells—so even more toxic chemicals! Softeners are made to stay in your clothes for

long periods of time. Chemicals are slowly released either into the air for you to inhale or onto your skin for you to absorb.

"Dangerous Pesticides in Your Hand Soap." Triclosan, the pesticide in personal care products. *Our Toxic Times,* June 12, 2009. Food and Water Watch. Kathy Dolan. wwwfoodandwaterwatch.org.

Triclosan is a dangerous pesticide lurking in most homes (soaps, facial cleansers, exfoliants, personal care products). In 2005, an FDA advisory panel of experts voted 11 to 1 that antibacterial soaps were no more effective than regular soap and (warm) water in fighting infections.(My note: I've read it's created a "superbug," resistant to germs and viruses.)

"Not Just a Pretty Face: The Ugly Side of the Beauty Industry." Stacy Malkan, co-founder of the Campaign for Safe Cosmetics and author of *Not Just a Pretty Face.* Sept. 12, 2013.

"When we tested products back in 2010, we found a number of allergens and hormone-disrupting chemicals in fragrances." The world's largest retailer, Walmart, will require (as of Sept. 12, 2013) companies to reduce or eliminate a priority list of hazardous chemicals from cosmetics, personal care items, and cleaning products sold in its stores. This is a huge victory for the millions of people who are demanding safer products. Large support organizations include: Campaign for Safe Cosmetics; Breast Cancer Fund; EWG (Environmental Working Group); Clean Water Action; Women's Voices for the Earth; Commonweal Friends of the Earth; Black Women for Wellness; Coming Clean; Teens Turning

Green; Cancer Schmancer; We Act for Environmental Justice; Story of Stuff plus; and others.

"A Toxic Tour of Your Bathroom?" Friends of the Earth, June 22, 2004. sierraclub.org.
When you use shampoo, deodorant, nail polish, aftershave, and other products on your body, you're exposing yourself to an array of untested chemicals, some of which have been linked to cancer, birth defects, and a variety of health problems. (EWG study of 7,500 + personal care products) Unfortunately, the U.S. government lets cosmetic companies use unlimited amounts of chemicals with no required testing, no monitoring of health effects, and inadequate labels.

"What's Lurking in Your Cosmetics and Toiletries?" (from "Children at Risk from Cosmetics," MN Kids Enviro Health, Severin Carrell, May 30, 2004. Children are at greater risk of cancers and fertility problems in later life because of the growing use of cosmetics and toiletries. Concern includes baby wipes, bubble baths, and parabens used as preservatives in body lotions like Johnson's Baby Soft Wash. (My note: Fragrances in these products compound the danger and problems.)

HOUSEHOLD CLEANERS

EWG's Hall of Shame—Toxins in the Home.
EWG's list of toxic household cleaners: Simple Green;
Spic & Span; Scrubbing Bubbles; Mop & Glo; Damp
Rid; Drano; Fume-Free Oven Cleaner (CVS); Glade;
Comet; Febreeze Air Effects (89 contaminants and is an
asthma trigger); Mr. Clean; Easy-Off Oven; 409; Lysol;
Fantastik; Clorox; Febreeze Sprays; Static Guard; Ajax;
Dynamo; Fab Ultra.

"8 Household Cleaning Agents to Avoid." Gaim Life
Staff. May 23, 2007. life.gaiam.com.
These affect the respiratory, nervous, and circulatory
systems. Irritants do liver and kidney damage.
Carcinogens. : chlorinated phenols, diethylene glycol,
phenols, nonylphenol ethoxylate, formaldehyde,
petroleum solvents, perchloroethylene, butyl cellosolve.
(My note: Research the products you are using.)

"Most Toxic Home Cleaning Products." Oct. 25, 2011.
www.thedailybeast.com.
List: Liquid Plumr (2); Tuff Stuff; Glass Plus; Lysol (3);
Legacy of Clean (4); Resolve (2); Bowl Fresh (3); Toilet
(2); Tough Stain.

"Safe Cleaning Tips for Your Home. EWG. Revised
Oct. 15, 2010.
Some safety tips for your family's health while you

clean: General— open windows; use gloves and other precautions; keep kids away; avoid "antibacterial"; never mix bleach with ammonia (or other chemicals), vinegar, or other acids; don't be fooled by labels; try natural alternatives like vinegar and baking soda; be careful with pine and citrus oil cleaners; avoid air fresheners. Kitchen/Bath—skip oven cleaners (biggest hazard); use baking soda and water paste and let it soak then scrub; avoid antibacterial soaps, harsh chemicals, fragranced products; use baking soda and vinegar; open windows to outside unless outside is polluted; use vinegar and water for mop water.

FOODS

"Acrylamide." American Cancer Society. Sept. 1, 2015. www.cancer.org.
Cooking at high temps causes a chemical reaction between certain sugars and an amino acid (asparagines) in the food, which forms acrylamide. Found highest in French fries and potato chips.

Chemical Cuisine: Do You REALLY Know What You're Eating? Dr. Gloria Gilbere. www.gloriagilbere.com or Amazon.com.
Outlines how chemicals in our food: cause weight gain; affect cognitive functions; are neurotoxins; add to total body burden; are responsible for most headaches (esp.

migraines); induce inflammation; and cause generalized multiple allergic responses. Dr. Gilbere is internationally respected as a natural health pioneer. She is best known for her groundbreaking book, *I Was Poisoned by My Body.*

EWG's Dirty Dozen Plus (from EWG's Shopper's Guide to Pesticides in Produce). 2015.
The following are most pesticide-contaminated, thus ones you might prefer to buy organic: apples, strawberries, grapes, celery, peaches, spinach, sweet bell peppers, imported nectarines, cucumbers, potatoes, cherry tomatoes, hot peppers. See the Clean Fifteen. (My note: I've also read a few times that carrots—or any fruit/veggie grown in or on the ground—have absorbed pesticides.

"Food Additives and Behavior." Jeremy Laurance, Health Editor. May 2004. news.independent.co.uk.
The impact of additives on the behavior of young children has been disputed since first claims in the 1940's that they caused fidgeting and inattention in children. Prof. John Warner, Dept. of Child Health at Southampton University, led a study and said, "These findings suggest that significant changes in children's hyperactive behavior could be produced by the removal of artificial colorings and sodium benzoate (preservative) from their diet." (My note: These two are still very much in use, as well as many more additives."

"Food Irradiation." RAD Town, USA, EPA. Feb. 23, 2015. www.epa.gov/radtown.
EPA says irradiation does not make food radioactive. (My note: How can it NOT be? It's exposed to unreal amounts of radiation, and workers at the facilities have to follow OSHA radiation protection rules. A friend who raised chickens said she heard the dead chicken vats were irradiated and used in nugget meals. I hope this is not true! I've eaten these. Have you?)

"Harmful If Swallowed—The Dangers of Food Irradiation." Dr. Gayle Eversole, PhD,ND. Nate Curtis. *Natural News ,*Sept. 1, 2013.
www.naturalnews.com041878.
These findings are similar to those of Dr. Mercola.com. In addition, food irradiation exposes food to the equivalent of 30 million chest x-rays. These foods have second-rate nutrition and a "counterfeit freshness." Irradiation is a quick-fix with long-term consequences.

Idaho Observer: " Aspartame-The World's Best Ant Poison." Jan Jensen. June 12, 2006.
Use of NutraSweet to get rid of carpenter ants.

"Is Sugar Really that Bad? 78 Ways Sugar Can Ruin Your Health." (Compilation of facts from medical journals and other scientific publications)
In 1700, average sugar consumption was 4 lbs. a year; by 1800, 18 lbs.; by 1900, 90 lbs. Daily total consumption should be 25 grams. Be careful of hidden

high fructose corn syrup. One can of soda alone almost exceeds that amount. Whole fruits should be limited and juices avoided. Best fruits for low fructose (sugar) consumption: lime, lemon, passion fruit, prune, apricot, cantaloupe, raspberry, Clementine, kiwi, blackberry, sweet and sour cherry, strawberry, pineapple, grapefruit, boysenberry, tangerine, and mandarin orange. Of 78 dangers of sugar listed, included are: suppressed immune system; hyperactivity and concentration difficulties; cancer (My note: Sugar feeds cancers.); rise in triglycerides and harmful cholesterol; kidney damage; weakened eyesight; negatively affects clarity of mind and growth hormones; contributes to diabetes, eczema, headaches, depression, constipation, tooth decay, aging process, and obesity; and can cause arthritis, asthma, and candidiasis.

"Most Dangerous Chips to Eat." Mercola.com, July 7, 2005.
Acrylamide is formed from a reaction of cooking certain sugars and food amino acids at high temps. Highest levels are Cape Cod Robust Russet and Kettle Chips. He suggests throwing out doughnuts, French fries, potato chips, and all sodas.

"Nuclear Lunch: The Dangers and Unknowns of Food Irradiation." www.mercola.com.
Beginning in 1986, FDA has given the "green light" to expose nearly our entire food supply to nuclear

irradiation. Citizen opposition, not government regulation, is helping keep irradiated food off the store shelves. Risks involved far outweigh the presumed "benefits." Food is irradiated using radioactive gamma sources which break up the molecular structure of the food, forming free radicals. Free radicals react with the food to create new chemical substances like benzene (known carcinogen), formic acid, formaldehyde, and quinines-harmful to human health. Irradiation destroys 20-80% of essential vitamins. Studies indicate health problems like possible chromosome damage, miscarriage, immunotoxicity, kidney disease and damage, cardiac thrombus, and future cancer development.

Our Toxic Times. "Avoiding Fragrance Chemicals as Indirect Food Additives." Jennifer Wilson, O.T.T., October 2006.
Superstore and supermarket foods frequently become contaminated by laundry detergent vapors and other scented products on the shelves. (My note: I KNOW this to be a fact! I've had to return even boxed foods because I could smell or taste fragrance or pesticide in the food I had purchased.)

"The Sugar Blues." Holly Holiman, RN, Health Coach. Jan. 5, 2016. hollyholiman.com/blog.   Sugar is bad for us for many reasons. A few reasons include: it promotes diabetes and obesity; suppresses our immune systems; leads to inflammation; worsens arthritis; increases cholesterol and triglycerides; makes us age faster; is addictive; and feeds cancer. Names for sugar include corn syrup, sucrose, fructose, dextrose, glucose, and lactose. Honey, agave, brown sugar, powdered sugar, turbinado sugar – it's all sugar! 1 of 11 Americans has diabetes; 1 of 3 pre-diabetes. The average American consumes 150 lbs of sugar a year, 38 tsp. a day. Recommended intake is 2 1/2 – 6 tsp. a day. It's important to replace sodas, fruit juices, and sport drinks with water, tea, and coffee. Look for cereal with five ingredients or less.

"Viral Adulteration of the U.S. Food Supply Gets FDA Approval." Byron J. Richards, CCN. Aug. 24, 2006. Newswithviews.com.
Live viruses will be sprayed on cold cuts, sausages, hot dogs, sliced turkey and chicken. FDA plans to use one infectious organism to fight another.

"Chemicals Have Replaced Bacteria and Virus as the Main Threat to Health." Dr. Dick Irwin, Toxicologist, Texas A & M University. July 26, 2012. www.lesstoxicguide.ca.

We are beginning to see, as the major cause of death in the latter part of the 20th century into the 21st century, diseases that are of chemical origin.

"Create a Safe and Healthy Home: Know Your ABC's." Dr. Joyce M. Woods and team. July 30, 2014.

Think of your home as a toxic waste dump. More than 72,000 synthetic chemicals have been produced since WWII—and the average home contains at least 62 of these toxic chemicals. An EPA survey concluded that indoor air is 2-5 times more polluted than outdoor air (paints, strippers, solvents, wood preservatives, aerosol sprays, cleaners and disinfectants, air fresheners, hobby supplies, dry-clean clothes, detergents, personal care items, etc.) The National Cancer Association listed household cleaners and detergents as the big reason cancer rates have almost doubled (that's from 1960 to 2004). Cancer is the #1 cause of death by illness for children. Since 1980, asthma has increased 600 %! The Canadian Lung Association identified household cleaners and cosmetics as the culprits. These chemicals have two primary points of entry— the skin and nose. The U.S.-Canadian Commission on Chemicals is trying to ban bleach in North America. (My note: Hydrogen peroxide is reputed to be its substitute.) It's being linked to the rise in breast cancer in women, reproductive problems in men, and learning/behavior problems in children. Chemicals are attracted to and stored in fatty tissue. The brain is a prime target because of its high fat content and rich blood supply. Air-out your house often with cross ventilation. Some diseases commonly related to chemical exposure include: fibromyalgia, chronic fatigue syndrome, arthritis, lupus, multiple sclerosis, Alzheimer's, Parkinson's, irritable bowel, depression, hormonal problems. (My note: This list has greatly expanded now, especially in the area of cancers.) In the USA in 2004, the #1 cause of accidental poisoning was Dawn dish detergent. Steam from our dryer vents is extremely toxic from chemicals in fabric softener sheets and residues from detergents and bleach.(My note: also steams from dishwashers, etc.) Research the ingredients in products you use.

"Environmental Exposure in Child Care Centers." Dr. A. Bradman, Center for Environmental Research and Children's Health. April 15, 2012. cerch.org.
Study finds elevated levels of formaldehyde and other contaminants in daycare centers. Researchers noted that children are more vulnerable than adults to environmental exposures and spend many hours a week in daycare.

"Environmental Illnesses in U.S. Kids Cost $76.6 billion in one year." Environmental News Service, May 4, 2011. www.ens.-newswire.com.
Three studies by Mt. Sinai scientists, published in the

May issue of *Health Affairs,* reveals the economic impact of toxic chemicals and air pollutants in the environment.

"Summary of Principles for Evaluating Health Risks in Children Associated with Exposure to Chemicals." European Public Health Alliance, 2006. www.epha.org. 351 page joint report from UN Environment Programme, World Health Organization, and International Labor Organization.
From conception through adolescence, rapid growth and developmental processes occur that can be disrupted by exposures to environmental chemicals.

Surgeon General: Second-hand Smoke Kills. "Second-hand Smoke Health Threat Worse than Believed." Marc Kaufman. *Washington Post,* June 28, 2006.
CDC reported in 2005 that second-hand smoke killed more than 3,000 nonsmokers from lung cancer, approximately 46,000 from coronary heart disease, and as many as 430 newborns from SIDS.

"Top 10 Unnecessary Toxic Products." Margie Kelly. Sept. 17, 2012. Care2.com.
Vinyl plastic; fragrance products; canned food; dirty cleaners; bottled water; lead lipstick; nonstick cookware; triclosan antibacterial agent; oil based paints; and finishers.

"Toxic Dreams: Crib Mattresses May Release Risky Fumes." Child Bedding, EWG. April, 2014. www.ewg.org.
Under the current law (Toxic Substances Control Act), it's nearly impossible to get toxic chemicals labeled and out of children's mattresses. University of Texas at Austin did a study of foam from 20 old and new crib mattresses. They found more than 30 VOC's released, some of which are linked to respiratory irritation and allergic reactions (phenol, fragrance, allergens, limonene, linalool). They also discovered that the sleep zone of the crib gave off the most intense VOC fumes. New cribs released four times as much as old cribs. These results are especially troubling because infants' respiratory systems are fragile, babies spend much of their first year in a crib, and body heat intensifies emissions.

"U.S. Facing 'Grievous Harm' from Chemicals in Air, Food, Water." *The Washington Post,* Lyndsey Layton. May 7, 2010. www.washingtonpost.com.
An expert panel that advises the President on cancer said Americans are facing "grievous harm" from chemicals in the air, food, and water that have largely gone unregulated and ignored. Children are particularly vulnerable because they are smaller and are developing faster than adults. (Check-out recent water source problem in Flint, MI.)

PESTICIDES

Children's Health Collection 2013: "Risk Factor for Childhood Brain Tumors." Julia R. Barrett. *Environmental Health Perspectives,* Nov. 2012. Epidemiologic data have suggested a link between pesticide exposures and childhood brain tumors.

Informed Choices for Healthier Living. www.wtv-zone.com/infchoice. Covington, LA.
It notes a woman who became very ill after pesticide and fertilize were spread on a golf course near her home. (My note: I've read of several occurrences similar to this.)

"Six Agrochemical Companies Indicted for Crimes against Humanity." Pesticide Action Network. UK, Nov. 16, 2011. www.pan.uk.org.
Big 6 (Monsanto, Dow, BASF, Bayer, Syngonta, and DuPont) accused of violating human rights by promoting reliance on the sale and use of pesticides known to undermine internationally recognized rights to health, livelihood, and life.

"Green Cleaner Required in Illinois Schools." Caryn Rousseau. Associated Press, May 15, 2008.
School uses just four (4) spray bottles for cleaning, filled with cleaners low on irritating chemicals and safer for students, staff, and the environment, rather than an array of harsh chemicals.

Greener School Cleaning Supplies. EWG, Nov. 3, 2009. www.ewg.org. Greener school cleaning supplies + fresh air and healthier kids.
New research links school air quality to school cleaning supplies. Among hundreds of chemicals identifiable in school cleaners were: 6 known to cause asthma (Childhood asthma has more than doubled since 1980, and, in 2009, 10% of children have it.) (My note: This number has increased.); 11 known, probable, or possible human carcinogens (Childhood cancer rose 28% from 1974 –1998.) (My note: And continues to rise.) ; 283 on which there's almost no scientific data. Some of the products tested are widely used in American households. Comet-disinfectant powder cleanser had 146 contaminants including formaldehyde (asthma), benzene, chloroform, and four other chemicals identified by CA as causing cancer or reproductive harm. Simple Green-93 chemicals, including two linked to cancer and one linked to cancer and asthma. Febreeze Air Effects-89 airborne contaminants including acetaldehyde (linked to cancer).

Healthy Schools Network, Inc: "What You Can Do at Your School." www.healthyschools.org.
Suspect that your child's school has indoor environmental problems when the roof leaks, it smells from being new or newly remodeled, it is fully carpeted, your child comes home sick or exhausted, an odor is clinging to clothes, he or she has health or learning problems only at school, the school has a damp or musty smell or recent water problems, or it uses toxic chemicals to prevent pests. (My note: Avoid strong, fragranced cleaning chemicals and the fragranced plug-ins or wall mounted deodorizers.)

"MN Lawmaker Wants Scent-Free Schools." Fox News, March 2008 and Martiga Lohn, *Star Tribune*, Mar. 10, 2008.
A fragrance-free educational campaign to discourage students from dousing themselves in scents that aggravate classmates with asthma and other health problems

ACKNOWLEDGMENTS

I first want to thank Jesus, the Great Physician, for helping me survive the throes of an illness caused by chemicals.

I thank my many friends for their encouragement and prayers during the four plus years it took to get this book finished. Special thanks to my critique group from Ozarks Chapter of American Christian Writers in Springfield, MO.

Joneen Copeland, I cannot thank you enough for the trips to my house and hours spent helping get *36 A DAY!* ready for publication. You also composed the perfect cover for this book! Joneen is also a writer. Among her publications are: <u>Character Tails: Diligence, Cooperation, & Patience</u>; <u>Have Patience! (¡Ten Paciencia!)</u>; <u>Anita la Hormiga Aprende Diligencia (Anita the Ant Learns Diligence)</u>; <u>Queenie's Transformation</u>; <u>Cristie Crab's Shopping Spree</u>; <u>Jasmine's Safari Adventure</u>. Available at Amazon.com.

Marilyn Collins (<u>Step-By-Step Writing Guides: Series 1-7</u>; <u>The Old Burying Ground: Beaufort, North Carolina</u>; <u>Rogers: The Town the Frisco Built</u>; and <u>Rogers, Arkansas)</u>, many thanks for editing my editing.

Dana Abrahamson, thank you for your personal contribution to *36 A DAY!* (pp. 79-86).

And I thank Amazon for making available to writers a venue for publishing works that spring forth from their hearts.

ENDNOTES

[i] Charlotte Gerson and Morton Walker, D.P.M. *The Gerson Therapy, Revised. The Proven Nutritional Program for Cancer and Other Illnesses* (New York, NY: Kensington Publishing Corp., 2001, 2006).

[ii] Julia Kendall, ref. Lance Wallace, EPA, "Sweet Poison: The Dangers of Perfume," (excerpts from MSDS Health Hazard Information), Oct. 16, 2003; 2015.

[iii] Carol Potera, "Scented Products Emit a Bouquet of VOC's," Environmental Health Perspectives, Jan. 1, 2011.

[iv] Fragrance: A Growing Health and Environmental Hazard, 1991 EPA study by Klaw Ferlow, May 2008.

[v] "Making Sense of Scents," Compiled by the late Julia Kendall, borrowing from Irene Wilkenfeld's "Fragrance Facts." ALSO IFRA (International Fragrance Assoc.)-in every sense.www.infraorg.org.

[vi] John P. Thomas, "Is Your Health Being Destroyed by Other People's Toxic Fragrances?" Health Impact News, June 9, 2014.

[vii] Dr. Joyce M. Woods and team, "Create a Safe and Healthy Home: Know Your ABC's," July 30, 2014. ALSO "Popular Shampoos Contain Toxic Chemicals Linked to Nerve Damage," Jan. 11, 2005.

[viii] "Dangerous Beauty: 5 Scariest Beauty Products." *Forbes,* March 12, 2012.

[ix] "Toxic Beauty Ingredients to Avoid." *Huffington Post. Nov. 12, 2013.*

[x] Dr. Anne C. Steinemann, Lisa G. Gallagher, Amy L. Davis, and Ian C. MacGregor, "Chemical Emissions from Residential Dryer Vents During Use of Fragranced Laundry Products," Springer Science and Business Media, *Air Quality, Atmosphere, and Health,.* March 1, 2013.

[xi] Class Action Lawsuit Against Fragrance Chemical Companies, Oct. 2012. Fragrance Free Warrior 328963298198 ALSO Air Freshener Class Action Lawsuit.

[xii] "New Study Finds Scented Candles and Air Fresheners Pose Dangerous Health Risks," Dec. 18, 2015. www.womansday.com/health.

[xiii] Mark Peplow, "Fears Raised as Plug-ins Linked to Cancer Compounds," (also: "Air Fresheners Cause a Stink.") May 10, 2004. ALSO "Ingredients in Deodorizers." Clinical Toxicology of Commercial Products. Gosselin, Smith, and Hodge, 1984. EPA, TSCA, Sect. 21, 2015.

[xiv] Vinegar, Better than Prescription Drugs? www.omaha.com, Sept. 25, 2014. ALSO Sanitize your Home Naturally Without Harmful Fumes. Greenopedia. Greenopedia.com/sanitize-naturally.

[xv] Pesticide-Induced Diseases: Alzheimer's,"Beyond Pesticides, www.beyondpesticides.org. ALSO 11 Commonly Used Pesticides Linked to Parkinson's and Alzheimer's. articles.mercola.com. Feb. 20, 2014.

[xvi] Informed Choices for Healthier Living. www.wtv-zone.com/infchoice. Covington, LA. ALSO Department of Health. 15 Pesticides. www.health.gov.au

[xvii] EHHI: The Harmful Effects of Vehicle Exhaust, www.ehhi.org/reports/exhaust. ALSO Cars, Trucks, & Air Pollution, Union of Concerned Scientists, www.ucsusa.org.

[xviii] Fragrance: A Growing Health and Environmental Hazard, 1991, EPA study by Klaw Ferlow, May 2008.

[xix] "Chemicals in Tobacco Smoke," Center for Disease Control and Prevention, (CDC), Mar. 21, 2011.

[xx] American Lung Association, "600 Ingredients in Cigarettes," www.lung.org.

[xxi] Dr. Frank Lipman, "20 Ways to Detox your Home, www.drfranklipman.com. May 14, 2012.

[xxii] Vaccines and Neurological Damage, Mercola.com. (Controversy in this area so do your research!)

[xxiii] Dr. Sanjay Gupta, OTC Drug Dangers You Should Know About, Everyday Health, www.everydayhealth.com. Mar. 20, 2014.

[xxiv] Johnson & Johnson: History, Products, Recalls, and Lawsuits, www.drugwatch.com/manufacturers, 2013.

xxv Katie Little, Fast Food Still Full of Additives, Even as Menus Simplify, CNBC, June 5, 2014.

xxvi Joyce Meyer, *New Day, New You,* Faith Words, New York, NY: Hachette Book Group, 2007, pg. 305.

xxvii Andrea Cespedes, What Kinds of Meat Do Fast-Food Places Use in their Burgers? Healthy Eating, 2013.

xxviii "Is Sugar Really that Bad? 78 Ways Sugar Can Ruin Your Health," (compilation of facts from medical journals and other scientific publications).

xxix Kobylewski, Sarah, PhD candidate, and C. Michael Jacobson, Executive Director CSPT, "Food Dyes: A Rainbow of Risks," News release from Center for Science in the Public Interest, June 29, 2010.

xxx "Food Additives to Avoid," EWG, www.ewg.org. ALSO Jeremy Laurance,"Food Additives and Behavior," Health Editor, May 2004, www.independent.co.uk.

xxxi *Idaho Observer, Jan Jensen,* "Aspartame-The World's Best Ant Poison," June 12, 2006.

xxxii "Lack of Drinking Water Deteriorates Human Body," April 16, 2015. www.medicaldaily.com.

xxxiii Sylvia Tremblay, MSc,"Consequences of Lack of Water," June 10, 2015.

xxxiv Honor Whiteman, "How Coca-Cola Affects Your Body When You Drink It," Aug. 15, 2015, www.medicalnewstoday.com. ALSO 6 Harmful Effects of Drinking Coke or Pepsi, www.healthy-drinks.net, Feb. 25, 2014.

xxxv Holly Holiman, RN, Health Coach, "The Sugar Blues," Jan. 5, 2016. hollyholiman.com. ALSO Kris Gunnars, BSc, How Food Addiction Works (and What To Do About It.) https://authoritynutrition.com, July 2015.

xxxvi The HOLY BIBLE, NIV, Grand Rapids, MI: Zondervan, 1990, pg. 1776.

xxxvii "Secret Chemicals Revealed in Celebrity Perfume, Teen Body Sprays," EWG, May 12, 2010, www.ewg.org.

xxxviii President's Cancer Panel: Environmentally Caused Cancers, (Also: "Grievous Harm-The Report of the President's Cancer Panel,") Environmental Health News, May 7, 2010-a 240 page report.

[xxxix] Guide to Less Toxic Products, Nova Scotia Allergy and Environmental Health Assoc.

[xl] CDC's Fragrance-Free Policy, Spring 2010. ALSO CDC-"Indoor Environmental Quality," Chemicals-Odors, Nov. 3, 2015, www.cdc.gov.

[xli] Gosselin, Smith, and Hodge,"Ingredients in Deodorizers," Clinical Toxicology of Commercial Products, 1984, EPA, TSCA, Sect. 21, 2015.

[xlii] Lysol, Ignorance, and The FDA, Project Accept.org, Oct. 5, 2014.

[xliii] EWG's Guide to Healthy Cleaning/Lysol Cleaner Ratings, www.ewg.org/guides.

[xliv] "Making Sense of Scents," Compiled by the late Julia Kendall, borrowing from IreneWilkenfeld's "Fragrance Facts," www.scentsforyouteam.com.

[xlv] Guide to Healthy Cleaning, EWG, www.ewg.org.